D1217963

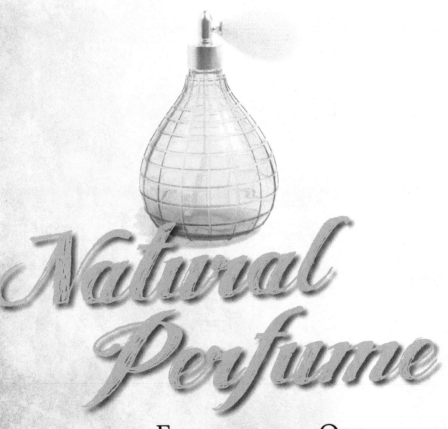

Natural Perfume

WITH ESSENTIAL OIL

Natural Perfume

WITH ESSENTIAL OIL

REBECCA PARK TOTILO

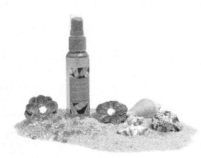

Natural Perfume with Essential Oil

Paperback ISBN: 978-0-9898280-9-3
Electronic ISBN: 978-0-9991865-0-3

Contents

CONTENTS

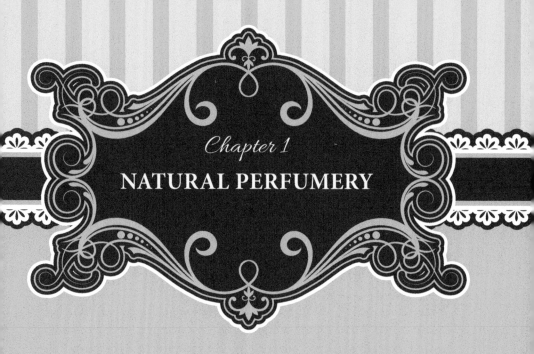

Chapter 1

NATURAL PERFUMERY

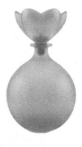

This will be the manner of the Kings...
he will take your daughters for perfumers...

— 1 SAMUEL 8:13-14

Creating natural perfumes with essential oils is as much an art as it is a science. Meticulously selecting each exquisite oil that nature provides such as rose, jasmine, or lime, then through systematic processes being able to transform these costly essences into a rich formula—a unique fragrance all on its own is truly amazing. The natural perfumer can then dilute this formula either with alcohol, waxes such as jojoba, beeswax, or a carrier oil such as coconut to create numerous products such as colognes, solid perfumes, body lotions, soaps, and more.

Using the same classic perfumery techniques and processes as mainstream houses, a natural perfumer can blend, dilute, age and bottle his or her own signature scent, rivaling any name brand.

"What many people don't realize is store-bought perfumes, whether Estee Lauder, Calvin Klein, or Ralph Lauren are made by one of seven mega-industrial fragrance houses. These houses, which are more like factory-style behemoths such as International Flavors & Fragrances (IFF), Givaudan, Firmenich, Quest, and Drom create and manufacture perfumes worldwide," according to John Berglund, founder of Tijon Parfumerie & Boutique.

What you won't find in a natural perfumer's organ are synthetic scents like banana or mango, although some artisans have creatively come up with ways to replicate these scents with tinctures. In addition, natural perfumers will use ambrette seed or another cruelty-free animal derivative in place of musk.

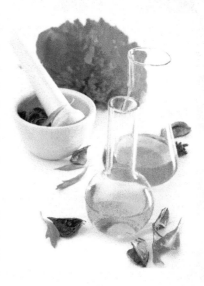

What you will find are essential oils and absolutes in every aromatic group or classification used in leading perfumeries (Floral, Green, Woods, and Oriental). From these, you can formulate a fragrance that is sophisticated, fresh, or seductive, depending upon your aspirational goal. The fragrance you formulate can be sophisticated, fresh, or seductive, depending upon the aspirational goal.

You can create natural fragrances that are subtle, giving you an aura of sweet bliss within your breathing space—only a few feet from your body. When you leave the room, your fragrance goes with you.

In this guide, you will discover how to create natural Eau de parfums that develop in layers, changing gradually with the chemistry of your skin. Working in unison with your body's chemistry, your fragrance gently evolves into your own signature scent, so you smell like you, not like everybody else. Discover how to create unique fragrances unlike anything on the market that will captivate your senses.

NATURAL VERSUS SYNTHETIC

According to the Natural Perfumers Guild, natural perfumery is defined as "the art of blending fragrance ingredients of natural origin to create aesthetically pleasing natural fragrance compounds used to fragrance a full range of industry products from fine perfume to personal and household products. The natural compound is the aromatic foundation for fragrant natural products and naturally fragranced products." [1]

*N*atural fragrances cannot ultimately be reduced to a formula because the very essences of which they are composed contain traces of other elements that cannot themselves be captured by formulas. [2]

– Mandy Aftel, Essence & Alchemy: A Natural History of Perfume

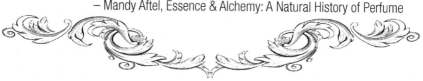

Perfumers have practiced their art for thousands of years, relying on nature for both inspiration and their source of materials. Due to demand and convenience, in the 1800s scientists began to separate natural raw materials into their component parts, isolating aroma chemicals. Within a few short years, they were able to duplicate these chemical constituents in a lab, resulting in the first synthetic perfumery ingredient.

Today, all mass-produced perfumes sold in large department stores contain synthetic manmade ingredients. Even if you see recognizable names on the label such as rose or carnation listed as an ingredient, it probably doesn't actually include real carnation or rose. Instead, typical synthetic replacements are used, which include chemical blends such as Phenylethylacohol 2 for rose and Methyl Diantillis 0.5 for carnation. Often these notes are derived from petrochemicals and may contain phthalates. The Environmental Working Group (EWG) reports they typically contain a dozen or more of potentially hazardous synthetic chemicals.

How many fragrances contain petrochemicals, you ask? On average, 80% of fragrance formulations are comprised of these chemicals and in some cases, up to 100% of the formula is synthetic. The worst part is, consumers may not even be aware of the contents in their favorite cologne, even when they've checked the label. The FDA allows these companies to withhold fragrance ingredients in order to protect trade secrets. According to Wendi Berger of the Pour le Monde parfums,[3] "this gives companies the freedom to load some fragrances with unknown chemicals, sensitizers, potential hormone disruptors and chemicals not assessed for safety."

These chemicals can be very dangerous to a person's health considering that 60% of what we put on our skin, the largest organ in our body, gets absorbed into the bloodstream. And, unfortunately, the liver and kidneys can't help filter these toxins; the skin is all on its own. The skin absorbs these chemicals in a few ways:

- By direct application.
- By contact with chemically-based items.
- By exposure to the air containing chemically-based fragrances.

Once these toxins accumulate in your body's organs, they can trigger allergic reactions, migraines, asthma attacks, nausea, eczema, and many other sensitivities.

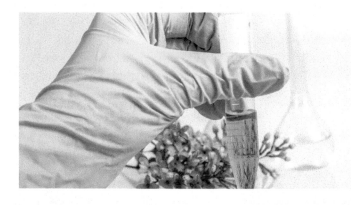

Some of the most talked about ingredients of concern in fragrances today include parabens, phthalates, and synthetic musks, according to Wendi Berger of Pour le Monde. "Parabens can interfere with the production and release of hormones while phthalates is a known carcinogen that can damage the liver and kidneys, cause birth defects, decrease sperm counts and cause early breast development in girls and boys. Studies now show that synthetic musks not only disrupt hormones, but traces have been found in fat tissue, breast milk, body fat, umbilical cord blood, both fresh and marine water samples, air, wastewater and sludge."

Today, there is a growing surge of consumers who want fragrances that contain only rich and complex natural ingredients. Fortunately for the natural perfumer, natural materials continue to be grown, processed and distributed and can create pleasing products that contain ingredients of natural origin to meet this demand.

Fragrance Ingredients of Natural Origin as defined by the Natural Perfumers Guild include:

1. Botanical raw materials, such as flowers, barks, seeds, leaves, twigs, roots, rinds, etc.
2. Exuded materials from plants, such as oleoresins, balsams, and gums.
3. Animal derivatives, such as ambergris and Hyraceum tinctures and absolutes, etc.
4. Soil products such as mitti and minerals such as amber.
5. Essential oils derived from natural raw materials by dry (destructive), steam, or water distillation or by mechanical processes, such as expressed or cold-pressed. Also included are other forms of essential oils, such as rectified oils, fractional distillations, molecular distillations, terpeneless oils, and folded oils.

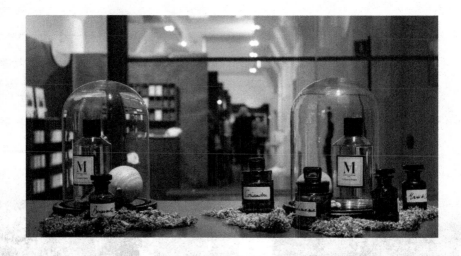

6. A natural isolate is a molecule removed/isolated from a natural fragrance material, as defined by the Guild, which contains the isolate. Processes that are acceptable for removing/ isolation are: fractional distillations, rectifications and molecular distillations of natural fragrance materials as defined by the Guild (exceeds ISO 9235).

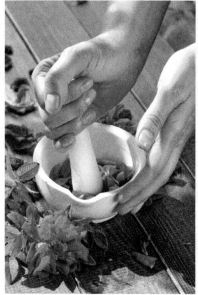

7. Other distillation products such as hydrolats (hydrosols, floral waters).

8. Tinctures derived by macerating a natural raw material in ethanol, such as tincture of vanilla.

9. Infusions obtained by macerating a natural raw material in a wax such as jojoba or a fixed oil such as almond oil.

10. Concretes, absolutes, and resinoids, all extracted from natural raw materials using a solvent other than water, followed by removal of the solvent by natural methods such as distillation/ evaporation. Solvents may include hexane, CO2, and others. Absolutes and pomades from enfleurage by the methods listed here.

11. Attars, rhus, and choyas.

12. A fragrant natural product is made by combining a natural fragrance compound with a wholly natural carrier. A fragrant natural product may be labeled "natural" (e.g. natural perfume, natural soap, natural massage oil, room spray, linen spray, etc.).

Associated products may include carriers that are used to deliver natural fragrance. Some carriers are pure and natural (such as ethanol from grain, sugar beets, grapes, or sugar cane; expressed oils; waxes, etc.), and

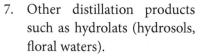

some are simple and partly or entirely synthetic (such as some specially denatured alcohols and silicone fluids). Some carriers can be wholly natural, partially or completely synthetic. [5]

As the natural perfumer, you know exactly what each bottle contains because you get to select the ingredients used personally. This can come in handy when creating a fragrance for a friend or family member who may suffer from chemical sensitivities and asthma. In most cases, they won't find natural ingredients bothersome like fragrances made with synthetics. Your natural perfumes will deliver healing instead.

RARE AND EXPENSIVE OILS

The drawback to using natural materials is, of course, they can be more expensive, simply because natural extracts may be scarce and difficult to source. Jasmine, for example, is priced at $226.00 for one ounce at the time of this writing. That's not to say some artificial perfumes don't contain pure essential oils, when they do. Typically this is a small percentage, though. While the mainstream perfume industry spends considerably less on aroma chemicals for their products, they do spend millions on marketing for a share in this $26 billion dollar industry. Natural perfumers will spend most of their budget on obtaining extravagant essences but are able to create smaller batches and experiment more.

WHAT MOTHER NATURE PROVIDES

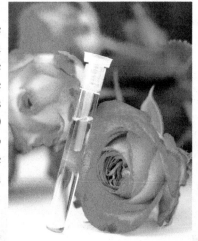

With numerous pure essential oils to choose from, there will still be scents missing from your perfume organ. For instance, notes like mango, banana and peach are impossible to extract from nature. Big perfume houses have access to a vast library of over 3,100 stock chemical ingredients (there are up to 10,000+ synthetic notes available), while the naturalist is limited to 300 notes from what Mother Earth provides.

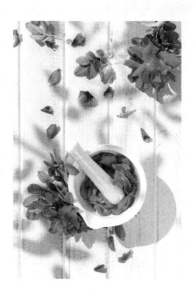

STAYING POWER

One of the biggest complaints about using natural ingredients in perfumes is that the scent doesn't last long on the skin. Natural perfumes generally do last two to three hours and then need to be reapplied to the skin at the wearer's discretion. No doubt, manmade synthetics have a stronger staying power due to chemical preservatives.

NATURAL PERFUMERY

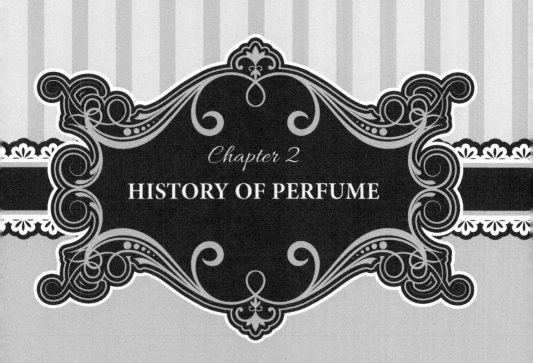

Chapter 2

HISTORY OF PERFUME

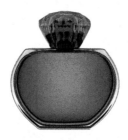

I anoint myself everyday with oil, burn perfumes and use cosmetics that make me worthier of worshipping thee.

– PRAYER TO GOD MARDUK BY BABYLONIAN KING NEBUCHADNEZZAR II WHO REIGNED CIRCA 605-562 BC

Historical records reveal that people's use of scents, aromas, fragrances, and essential oils have been used in almost every culture for millenniums. The earliest evidence of the usage of essential oils occurred between 3000-2500 BC. Archeological evidence dating as far back as the Neolithic Stone Age almost 10,000 years ago offers insight into perfume's beginnings. One of the oldest discoveries to date is of fossilized resins found in Central China. The charred gum suggests that the resins were burned, most likely for religious purposes. During rituals, priests anointed their ceremonial robes with oil and burned incense. By the time of the Song Dynasty (AD 960-1279), the art of incense had become such a celebrated pastime that buildings included rooms specially designated for incense ceremonies.

Like China, India has used essential oils and resins for centuries and has been a core element of Ayurvedic medicine. "No one is sure how long Ayurvedic medicine has been practiced, possibly 4,000 years. Ayurvedic literature from 2000 BC records Indian doctors administering oils of

cinnamon, ginger, myrrh, coriander, spikenard and sandalwood to their patients," says Lorene Davies, founder of Essential Oil Academy. [6]

Both the Assyrians and Egyptians used scented essences as well. The ancient Egyptians held perfume right at the heart of their society. Incense was burned in sacrifice to their gods and perfumed oils were used to anoint and embalm their dead. During the excavations of tombs in the Valley of the Kings, there are recordings of countless finds of alabaster jars containing frankincense and myrrh. Cleopatra, the Queen of Egypt, drenched the sails of her ships with the most exotic fragrant essential oils so that their essences would herald her arrival along the banks of the Nile.

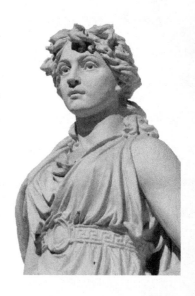

The Greeks attributed sweet aromas to their gods as well by burning incense. The ancient Greeks had a particular penchant for their perfumes and their myths and legends are full of the powers they bestowed on the oils. Circe entrapped Odysseus with a sacred perfume and the beguiling powers of Helen of Troy were attributed to a perfume gifted by Aphrodite.

The Babylonians perfumed the mortar with which they built their temples while the Hebrews scattered fresh leaves, twigs, and stems of fresh mint, marjoram and other herbs on the dirt floors of their homes and synagogues. By walking on these herbs, the fragrant essential oils would be released into the air. This practice was also common in the temple where they sacrificed animals so that the scent acted as a disinfectant as well as an air freshener.

Both Old and New Testaments of the Bible are full of references to aromatic resins, oils, and incenses enlightening the reader to their value in trade. Frankincense, for instance, was considered more valuable than gold during the time of Christ. By New Testament times, perfume took center stage in reflecting a person's status with its use. Mary, the

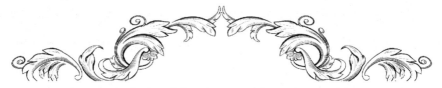

Since the beginning of time, immemorial man has used fragrances for religious, social and political occasions. Often in a crude form, other times in the form of incense, scent has played an invaluable part in how humans relate not only to one another but with their gods.

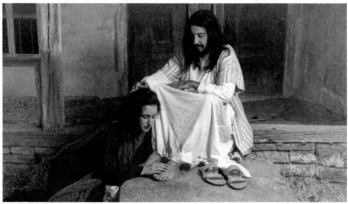

sister of Lazarus, washed the feet of Jesus with the fragrant oil of Nard (known today as spikenard) before his crucifixion. Essential oils were also considered medicine which was illustrated in the parable Jesus told about the Good Samaritan.

The Greek Hippocrates spoke highly of fragrances as did his contemporary Galen. Hippocrates, today considered the father of modern medicine, said, "The way to health is to have an aromatic bath and scented massage every day."

Both the Assyrians and Egyptians used scented oils. Because of this, the demand for the raw materials necessary to produce both fragrances and remedies led to the discovery of new ways to extract scents from the plants used. Such techniques as pressing, decoction, pulverization and maceration were developed and mastered by both the Assyrians and the Egyptians. They even made attempts to produce essential oils by distillation. It was not until the discovery of the writings of Arab Avicenna dating AD 790 that we see references to distillation. While it is unclear whether Avicenna discovered the process of distillation, his work contained diagrams of the required equipment for distilling plant materials.

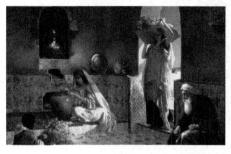

Slowly, the use of perfumes spread to Greece where they were not only used in religious ceremonies, but for personal purposes as well. When the Romans saw what the Greeks were doing, they began to use fragrances even more lavishly. Many manuscripts tell how herbs were brought from all over the world to produce the fragrances they used.

After the Roman Empire had fallen, the use of aromas for personal consumption declined. By medieval times most great houses in Europe still had rooms for private distillery, but the Catholic Church denounced the use of aromatics for personal use. Perfumes were instead reserved for use during religious ceremonies and to cover the stench of disease and death which abounded at that time. It wasn't until the Crusaders returned with exotic spices, gums, and resins from overseas that a new passion for scents exploded.

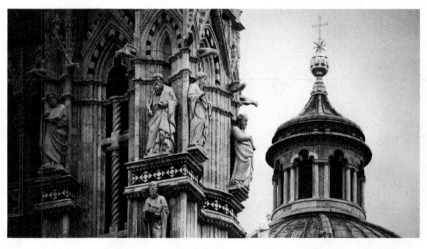

THE ANCIENT USES OF PERFUMES

In ancient times, essential oils and other aromatics were used for religious rituals, as well as for emotional and spiritual needs. According to the *Essential Oils Desk Reference* compiled by Essence Science Publishing, "Records dating back to 4500 BC describes the use of balsamic substances with aromatic properties for religious rituals and medical applications. The translation of ancient papyrus found in the Temple of Edfu, located on the west bank of the Nile reveals perfume recipes used by the alchemist and high priest in blending aromatic substances for rituals performed in the temples and pyramids. As well, Hieroglyphics on the walls of Egyptian temples depict the blending of oils and describe hundreds of oil recipes. These writings tell of scented barks, resins of spices, and aromatic vinegars, wines, and beers that were used in rituals, temples, for embalming and medicine. Thus, the Egyptians were credited as the first to discover the potential of fragrance and were considered masters in using essential oils and other aromatics in the embalming process. They created various aromatic blends for personal use, placing them in alabaster jars—a vessel specially carved and shaped for holding fragrant oils. In 1922, when King Tut's tomb was opened, 350 liters of oils were discovered in alabaster jars. Amazingly, because of the solidification of plant waxes sealing the opening of the jars, the liquefied oil was in perfect condition.

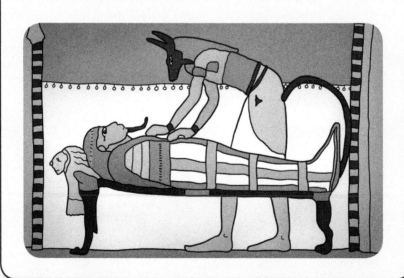

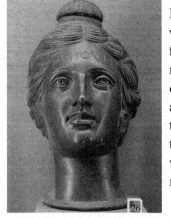

During the thirteenth century when trade with the Orient was reestablished, exotic flowers, herbs, and spices became more readily available around Europe. Venice quickly became the center of perfume trade and it was not long before perfumery spread to other European countries. The perfume trade continued to flourish even further when those returning from the Crusades reintroduced perfume for personal use.

At the same time, raw materials were being supplied to French perfumers by large flower-growing districts in the south of France. In 1370, Queen Elizabeth of Hungary commissioned her own fragrance, which was to change the face of perfume as we knew it. Hungary Water, as it came to be known, was the first blend to use alcohol. Comprised of rosemary, thyme, and brandy, the scent was to be worn and also consumed.

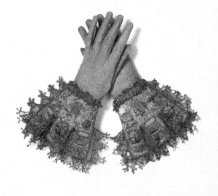

Meanwhile, in Italy, the arts began to flourish. By the 1500s, the Renaissance was at its very height and perfumery was an opulent expression of grace. In France, Henry II took a wife, Catherine de Medici, a formidable Italian noblewoman. During her younger years, Catherine had been given a pair of gloves. While the soft leather gloves were beautiful, their creator Guillamard, a tanner, disguised the stench of the tanning process scenting them with musk and ambergris. The effect was stunning.

Catherine took this idea home with her to Grasse where she established a business making these beautifully scented gloves. The industry became a powerhouse with recipes being carefully guarded secrets. So treasured were they, the rooms of her head perfumer Rene le Florentin were connected to Catherine's bedroom by a narrow corridor. Since the climate there lent itself beautifully to the cultivation of crops producing products such as amber, frangipani, jasmine and musk, Grasse provided scented gloves to appeal to the aristocracy across their land and beyond.

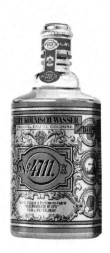

Fragrance had France in its grips. Louis XIV relished his "Perfumed Court:" furniture, clothes and even fans were scented to pervade a bouquet. By the eighteenth century, it reached maddening proportions. Records show that two quarts of Violet Cologne were delivered to Napoleon every week. It was even said that sixty years after the death of Josephine, her boudoir still reeked of the musk she had so adored.

Industry in Grasse flourished right up until the American Revolution made a trade in gloves no longer tenable. Despite this, the industry still had a sustainable resource in the knowledge they had gathered about perfumery. In 1789, Grasse produced its last pair of gloves and its first flacon of oil.

Meanwhile in Germany in 1709, a perfumer by the name of Giovanni Maria Farina created a blend which he called Eau de Cologne. The Italian

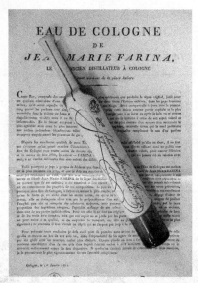

wrote to his brother, "I have found a fragrance that reminds me of an Italian spring morning, of mountain daffodils and orange blossoms after the rain," and he named it after his adopted hometown of Cologne.

Farina's blend of so many "nano-essences" was seen as a sensation and vials of the concoction were delivered to the royal houses. In 1806, the great grandson of Farina opened a perfumery business in the heart of Paris. The company that was later sold to Roger and Gallet now owns the rights to Eau de Cologne le vielle. The term *eau de cologne* is now used as a generic term for any fragrance that contains 2-5% concentration of essential oils in alcohol.

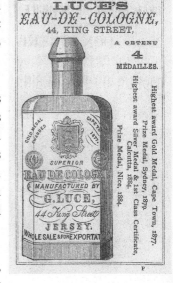

Across the Atlantic, in 1808 America's Florida Water was launched. Two centuries later, the scent is still in production. Based on Eau de Cologne, it contains fresh citrus head notes of bergamot, lemon, and neroli. Spicy notes of clove and cinnamon warm the mix, and it is finished with a floral accent of jasmine and rose.

As the twentieth century dawned, perfumes became the stock of trade for fashion houses and some of the greatest fragrances of our time were introduced to the market.

The family of Jean Francois Houbigants had been producing fragrances in Grasse since the eighteenth century. His scents were much sought after by the great and the good; his perfumes graced the homes of Napoleon and Alexander III. It is reputed that Marie Antoinette, fleeing Versailles disguised, was recognized by her scent as only royalty could afford fragrance from the House of Houbigants.

In 1912, Houbigants requisitioned the services of perfumer Robert Bienaimé to create Quelque Fleurs. It utilized his discovery of an element found in tonka beans called coumarins to create a whole new lighter fragrance. It was the first floral aldehydic fragrance and is reputed to have been the inspiration behind Chanel No. 5.

The recipe for Quelque Fleurs has never been published but had been reintroduced with slightly differing ingredients twice since. In total, it incorporates an astonishing 250 raw elements and requires 15,000 flowers to produce.

The heart of the fragrance is that of the spicy floral of carnation. It opens up with orange blossom and green notes of tarragon, bergamot, and lemon. Floral middle notes of iris, heliotrope and rose give way to the hay-like tonka bean, amber, civet, and musk. Despite its floral aroma, this has non-conformist depths. Quelque Fleurs was the chosen scent of radicals like Sarah Bernhardt.

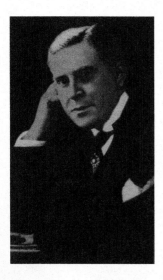

Coty's iconic powdery scent of Chypre was launched in the midst of the Great War. In 1908, Francois Coty acquired the manufacturing headquarters to Suresnes, near Paris. The colossal factory "La Cité des Parfum" employed 9,000 staff and made 100,000 bottles of perfume a day.

During the desolation of wartime, Coty wanted to embody his vision of love and beauty. The fragrance created has a striking but fleeting and haunting effect. Named after the island of Cyprus, the birthplace of Venus, the goddess of beauty and love, Chypre was a work of perfumery genius.

Coty reconstructed the much-loved blend of moss, bergamot, and labdanum of Roman times and added to them to give them a more modern edge. He mixed leathery notes to take off the sharpness of the notes then softened it with jasmine and lily of the valley as heart notes.

After the World War I, the production of the fragrance industry skyrocketed. US soldiers wanting to take home gifts to their loved ones lined Coty's pockets to a startling degree. By 1929, Coty was named as one of France's wealthiest men, his fortune amassed to over $34 million.

Gabrielle "Coco" Chanel spoke out to a whole new generation of flappers in 1921 when she commissioned Ernest Beaux to create No. 5. She felt that neither heady nor floral perfumes popular at the time spoke to the newly liberated women.

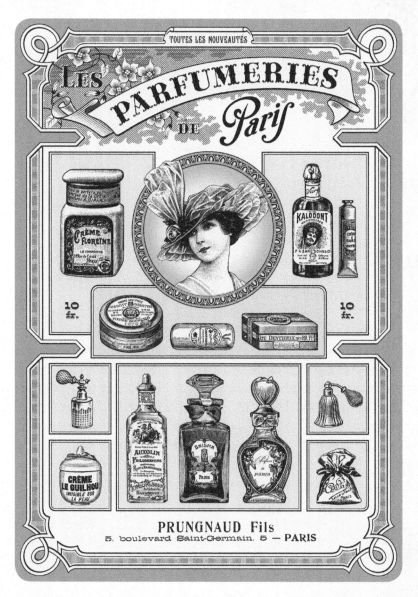

By late nineteenth century, synthetic materials for perfumes were being produced, which led to the beginning of perfumery in the modern age. With the introduction of synthetics, perfumes would no longer be exclusively used by the rich and famous. Now with synthetics readily available to produce perfumes, they could be made on a much larger scale, along with natural oils to help soften the synthetics. Today, natural products remain a critical part of the production of perfumes in modern formulations.

Beaux was well-known at the time for his experimentation using aldehydes in a fragrance, having been inspired by Quelque Fleurs. In No. 5, the aldehydes are overdosed giving the fragrance its familiar edge. The top notes of bergamot, lemon, and neroli made way for the heart notes of jasmine, rose, lily of the valley and iris. The lingering base notes of vetiver, sandalwood, amber and patchouli give it a lovely, sultry edge.

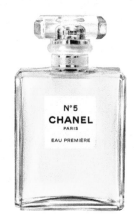

The bottle was part of the magic in the creation as much as the perfume. Chanel felt that the beautiful bottles of the past were not relevant to a fragrance made for the more liberated woman. Instead, she produced "pure transparency, an invisible bottle."

The number five was of particular significance to Chanel. As a child brought up in a convent, she noticed that the number five spoke to her over and over again. Five paths lead her to the cathedral each day, the grounds surrounding her home were covered with cistus, a five-petal flower. Recalling that she always showed her new collections on the fifth day of the fifth month, Chanel found significance in her choice of the fifth vial out of 12 bottles of perfume produced by Beaux. And so, No. 5 was born.

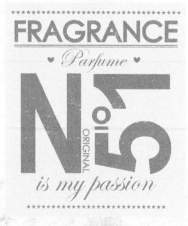

In the same year, Guerlain was creating a perfume of a very different type: the dark, heavy and exotic fragrance of Shalimar. Legend has it that Guerlain experimented with vanillin, pouring it straight into a bottle of Jinky, and the result was this magical concoction.

Guerlain had always considered vanilla to be an incredible aphrodisiac ingredient. The effect, when blended with the hay-scented coumarins of tonka bean, was electric. At the very top of the blend is the fresh sharpness of bergamot underlined with the thick aroma of opoponax, making it a truly seductive blend. On discovering his fellow countryman's interpretation of the oriental blend, Ernest Beaux was reputed to have cried, "If I do vanilla, I get Crème Anglais, when Guerlain does vanilla he gets Shalimar!"

The name Shalimar was taken from the gardens of the same name at the Taj Mahal, meaning Temple of Love. Disaster struck the company, though, when a rival company quickly launched a fragrance by the same name. During a long legal battle, the export bottles of Guerlain's products were labeled No. 90, its catalog number.

In 1925, when litigations were complete, Shalimar was rereleased and this time packaged in a stunning bottle designed by Raymond Guerlain and produced by Cristalleries de Baccarat. Exhibited in the decorative arts exhibition as an antidote to the Great Depression, the product took the world by storm.

Two years later in 1927, André Fraysse was asked to create a fragrance for the house of Lavin. As a gift to the 13-year-old daughter of the owner of the house for her birthday, she was asked to give it a name. On experiencing how the notes played out alternately, she was reminded of her love of music and arpeggio. The top notes of bergamot, peach, orange blossom, honeysuckle, and orris danced with the heart notes of rose, jasmine, coriander, and ylang ylang. Finally, base notes of sandalwood, vetiver, patchouli, vanilla and musk took the turn; the dance of the alternating notes of the perfume was called Arpege.

The year 1929 saw the release of Joy by Jean Patou. Designed by Henri Almeras, it was called "the most expensive perfume ever made." The floral scent was created as a reaction to the Wall Street crash which had snuffed out the fortunes of so many of the clientele of Patou's fashion house. Despite its high price tag, customers rushed to buy the scent in droves.

The secret of its success was the opulence of the scent. A stunning 10,000 jasmine flowers and 28 dozen roses were blended with ylang ylang, michelia, and tuberose to make just 30 milliliters of Joy. The strapline of its sales said that Joy brought the platonic idea of a flower rather than its earthly manifestation. Later in 2000, Joy was voted scent of the century.

In Europe, when war broke out, the role of women started to be seen in a different way. Just as the Great War gave birth to the flappers and scents like No. 5, the Second World War brought about her own fragrances.

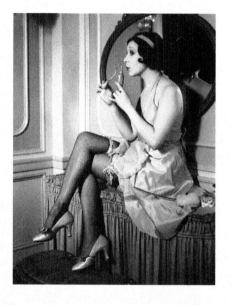

Designed in 1943 and launched in 1944, Rochas Femme embodied the decadence of the later years of the war. Inspired by heroines like Mae West, Edmond Roudnitska created a fragrance to portray the ripeness on the edge of decay. The fresh aldehydes opened up to an overripe plum tinged with violet, then musty patchouli and oakmoss to tinge the scent. Finally, the animal magnetism of civet and musk grasp the wearer, just as the passion of the moment.

During the hopeful days of peacetime, 1947 saw the introduction of Vent Vert. Its fresh outdoor sunshine vibration was the perfect match for the resurgence of femininity for that age. The career of Pierre Balmain was already riding the crest of a wave after the development (alongside Christian Dior) of the New Look dresses of the time. Gone were the waspish waists and stiff shoulders; in came in anbodices and excessive amounts of fabric in the skirts.

That year at the Cannes Film Festival, Vent Vert was offered to the public. The top notes of lemon, bergamot, key lime, neroli and basil explode with the fizz of a champagne cork and the freshness of sea spray. Even the

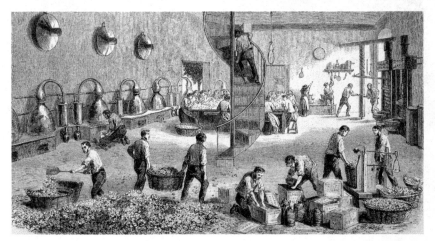

heart notes of Vent Vert are green. Galbanum, the spiciness of marigold, rose hyacinth and lily of the valley are reminiscent of a spring woodland. Underlining them all are the woody notes of oakmoss, sandalwood, and cedar. Vent Vert truly did embody the wind of change.

Lair Du Temps was designed by Robert Ricci as a celebration of the newly liberated generation of women. Rather than using the heady scents that had been so popular during the war, this product was designed to be the absolutely contrasting atmosphere of lightness and floating. Like the clothes of the period, the fragrance was expected to adapt to the personality of the wearer.

The magic of the fragrance really came to life when a colleague suggested adding benzyl salicylate to take on the floral edges from the carnation, violet, and rosewood. To crown the celebration, Ricci commissioned celebrated glassmaker Lalique to create a flacon topped with a pair of doves, symbols of the world's hope for peace.

Estée Lauder released her brilliant bath oil doubling as the fragrance Youth Dew in 1953. While women were putting a dab of other scents behind their ears, wearers of Josephine Catapano's creation were pouring literally bath loads down the drain.

The scent worked so well because it was very heavy, the notes becoming lighter in the dilution of the bath. Also, the product was incredibly essential oil laden. Top notes of aldehydes, shot through with orange, peach, bergamot and lavender, give it a richly sweet feeling. The heart then offers up cinnamon, cassia, orchid, jasmine, cloves, ylang ylang, rose, lily of the valley, and spices. The heavy base notes of tolu balsam, Peru balsam, amber, patchouli, musk, vanilla, oakmoss, vetiver and incense anchor this super sweet scent.

In its first year, Youth Dew sold 150,000 bottles of bath oil; by 1984, that number had grown to 150 million.

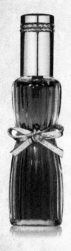

The fifties finally burned their pretty girl selves out, and the hippy movement began to take its place. Eau Neuve was released from the house of Lubin in 1968 with its fresh scent that completely embodied the flower power movement. It is said a fresh breeze pervades that brings in citrus notes. Orange, lemon, bergamot, thyme, chamomile, marjoram and lavender give the blend a light and floaty top note. Rose, jasmine, patchouli and oakmoss are melded with woody base notes that linger long after the initial notes have passed.

Interestingly, though, perhaps the wearer had a little clue that the radical scent for the new age was actually a reference to a far older scent. Rewind almost 200 years and Lubin released Eau de Lubin. The fragrance was an eau de toilette worn by Josephine and the last Queen Amelie. Somehow there seems to be cruel irony in that the nation who wanted so much to be revolutionary had no idea of its antiquated ties.

So now that brings us close to the present day. Perfumery still continues to be the largest industry in the area of Grasse and globally literally thousands of new scents are released every year. Discoveries into new methods continue to be made, and of course, marketing grows exponentially in our technological age. One can only wonder what the next 100 years will bring.

Chapter 3

THE NOSE KNOWS

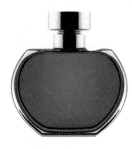

Perfume, that conqueror of the most subtle of our senses, that informer of our unspoken desires, perfume which from out of the unreliable depths of human memory uncovers the found of tears, the secret of pleasure.

– Colette

Our world is immersed in scent, yet with today's hectic pace, are we really aware of how big a part scent plays in our lives? How many times has a fleeting fragrance passed you by?

For some, scent is something to notice only in passing. Often, if the intensity is too great, we note this with some discomfort. But for many, scent is an accent to our day—a punctuation mark that energizes, lifts the mood and brings details into sharper focus. Of course, there is much science behind this too: the science upon which the ancient practice of aromatherapy is based.

Let's consider a typical day in the life of one who finds scents to be an indispensable part of her existence – we'll call it:

"A Scented Day in the Life"

The day begins with waking. Morning smells of coffee and the perfume of dewy wildflowers in the garden waft in on the breeze.

The intense aroma of freesia blooms rides in on rays of sunshine, bringing a half-waking euphoria as she begins her day.

Lavender-scented soaps and the unmistakable aroma of ylang ylang in her hair products both calm and invigorate, casting a rosy glow on the day ahead. On her skin, she uses a rich emollient cream infused with lemon verbena. It moisturizes and revitalizes her with a scent that is delicate and uplifting. It quickly disappears as it is absorbed into the skin, with a lingering yet subtle citrus freshness.

As she prepares for her busy day, she chooses an aromatherapy necklace to wear, placing a couple of drops each of rosemary, peppermint, and orange essential oils into the locket to promote focus and energy. No matter what the day might bring, this scent will be with her through every challenge, helping her to bring clarity to the tasks at hand.

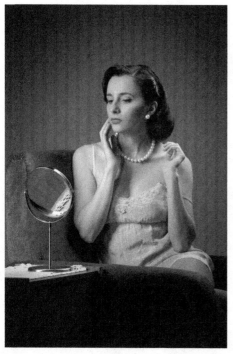

Walking to work, many more scents drift by on her passing: a rose bush in full bloom coaxes a smile, a gardenia brings thoughts of romance. As she enters her favorite café, she catches a tangy, woodsy scent on a man who passes close as she enters, evoking thoughts of mountain streams and the great outdoors. Her beverage is a highly scented Earl Grey tea, the spicy, tangy citrus aromas of bergamot motivates and revitalizes.

Arriving at the office, her senses are assailed with

a hundred scents at once: heavily perfumed men and women wearing every type of scent possible, from the sultry florals of the ladies to the pungent and spicy colognes favored by youth to the masculine, earthy notes of her male colleagues.

Making her way to her desk, something unknown activates an allergic response and her sinuses quickly begin to inflame. Luckily, she has a bottle of pure peppermint essential oil in her desk: placing a couple of drops in the palm of her hand, she brings it to her face and inhales sharply, feeling her airways clear immediately and leaving a tingling sense of freshness on the back of her palate.

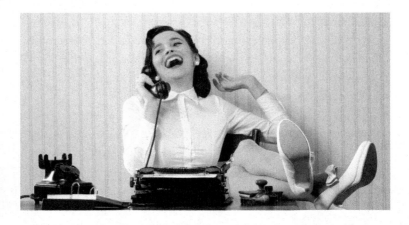

Her busy day is made easy by the subtle, permeating scent offered up by her aromatherapy necklace—the essential oil blend helps to keep her mind on track while enjoying the mingling of its pleasant, tangy and savory notes.

At lunchtime, she emerges back into a riot of fragrance, made doubly chaotic by the mad rush of people running in every direction. She chooses a spot outside in the park to enjoy her midday meal, taking in the smells of fresh-cut grass, damp earth, and the nearby flower beds, bursting with the heady fragrance of jasmine, rose, primrose, mock orange, and lilies. When it's time to return to work, these scents linger on in sweet memory as she readies to dive back into her daily tasks.

Aided by the focus-oriented essential oil blend she wears close, her phone conversations are productive and to the point, her afternoon presentation is concise and well-received, and she feels confident and accomplished as she tidies her desk, getting ready to leave. She thinks about the evening ahead: meeting coworkers for drinks at their local bistro, then back home to prepare for a date with that special someone.

The bar is crowded, and her nostrils are immediately assailed with food aromas and fading perfumery. She orders a gin cocktail infused with lavender and juniper berries, drinking in the scents as she sips, finding instant relaxation in the company of good friends. Soon, it is time to head home to get ready for her date.

The twilit rooms of her abode offer a quiet serenity, and she diffuses her own special blend of essential oils to induce calm: a drop or two each of frankincense, vetiver, chamomile, orange and rose calms her nerves and helps to balance her energies as it eases the butterflies. Not that she is nervous—well, maybe a little bit. It's the third date with a very special someone, and though she is looking forward to it, there is a tinge of anxiety to her thoughts. Everything must be just right—from her hair to her outfit to her scent.

A long, luxurious bath with a joyful blend of Roman chamomile, coriander seed, jasmine, ylang ylang, and geranium essential oils help to fill her heart with optimism as she soaks away the cares of the day. As she pats dry, subtle florals linger on her skin, seeming almost to emanate from her healthy inner glow.

Her closet is hung with packets of patchouli, lending a subtle, earthy note to her dress as she whisks it off the hanger. Dressing with care, she mists her hair with argan oil; lightly scented with rosemary, it provides a luxuriant shine from roots to tips. To complete the picture, she chooses a scent that is at once seductive and alluring: a heady blend of neroli, jasmine, patchouli, and vetiver. She dilutes it in almond oil and smooths it on her arms and legs, the carrier oil disappearing into the skin and leaving only subtle traces behind—and subtlety is precisely what she's after. Her scent will only be noticeable when someone is close enough to touch.

When they meet, he has brought her favorite flowers: a fragrant bouquet of lily of the valley, freesia, and yellow roses. Their night out is sweet and delicious, and she revels in his scent: an earthy, spicy blend of patchouli, sage, and oakmoss that lingers long into the night, even after they part.

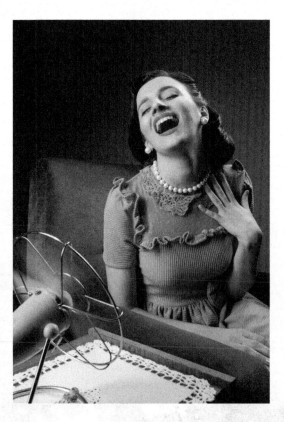

As the moon rises and the time for sleep draws near, she mists her pillows with sweet lavender to help lull her into a deep sleep, all the better to dream of the day's magic and that which is yet to come.

Did you know that just smelling the fragrance of a rose can bring healing and elevate your mood? Even when the scent is too faint to notice, healing is taking place. The sense of smell facilitated through the olfactory nerve invites the fragrance of essential oils into individual regions of the brain, enabling the body to process them naturally. The scent has the ability to stimulate the limbic region of the brain, pineal gland, and the pituitary gland.

The nose, which is wired differently than the other four senses, carries molecules directly into the emotional center of the brain where traumatic memories are stored. Essential oils become a vehicle by which repressed emotions can be released. Research has proven that these aromatic compounds can wield significant effects on the brain, in particular on the hypothalamus (the hormone command center of the body) and the limbic system (the seat of emotions).

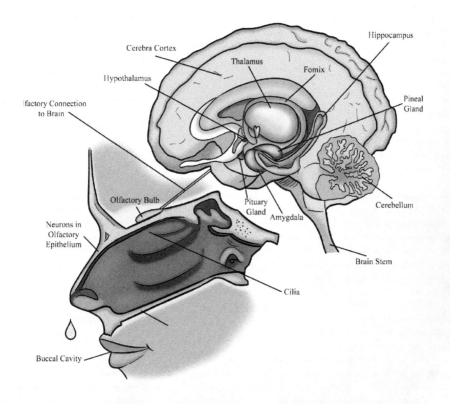

Olfaction, also referred to as "the sense of smell," is among the earliest of the human senses to arise during the evolution of man. The nerve endings in the roof of the nose receive smells emanating from people, objects, and animals, and converts them into electrical impulses that are then relayed to the olfactory bulb located in the forebrain. Some impulses are transmitted to the limbic system and are responsible for evoking emotions that are in line with the presenting situation. For example, one can detect food, enemies or a potential mate. Nice smells elicit pleasure from our bodies while repugnant smells raise the alarm in our bodies.

Information relayed to the limbic system is checked against any existing memory and identification of the scent is made. This also elicits the emotion that the given smell is usually associated with.

Of the five human senses, the sense of smell is the only one that is directly connected to the brain. The olfactory system, which is closely linked to the limbic system, has a vast influence on the body's physiology, while

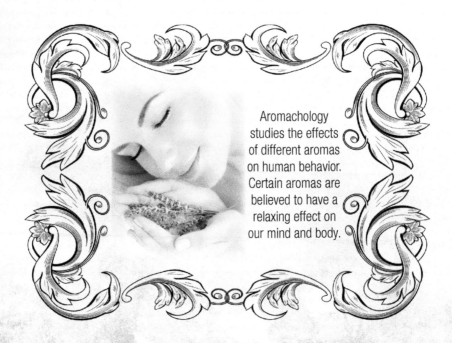

Aromachology studies the effects of different aromas on human behavior. Certain aromas are believed to have a relaxing effect on our mind and body.

the limbic system serves as the center for the human sex drive, memory, emotions, and physical drive.

Research now supports that essential oils have the ability to pass through the blood-brain barrier and stimulate various constituents of the brain. Their effect is quick and results in the relief of pain, promotion of sleep and if adrenaline release is stirred, the body is stimulated into an alert state. This knowledge has been used to treat various conditions such as sleep disorders and anxiety, and to provide relief from chronic pain.

FRAGRANCES IMPACT ON MOOD

When essential oils are diffused in the air, the oils reach the brain by means of the olfactory system. The olfactory membranes, with almost 800 million nerve endings, receive the micro-fine, vaporized oil particles and carry them along the axon of the nerve fibers, connecting them with the secondary neurons in the olfactory bulb. Impulses are then transported to the limbic system and the olfactory sensory center at the base of the brain. They then pass between the pituitary and pineal gland and move to the amygdala—the memory center for fear and trauma. The impulses travel to the gustatory center where the sensation of taste is perceived.

The olfactory, which is responsible for odor detection, sends impulses created by various odors to the amygdala. According to the WiseChoiceLiving.com website, the discovery that the amygdala plays a significant role in the storing and releasing of emotional trauma wasn't discovered until 1989, and ONLY odor or fragrance stimulation has a profound effect in triggering a response with this gland.

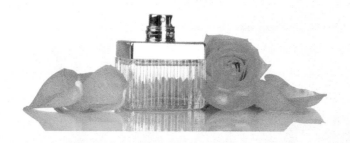

The limbic system, which is directly linked to those areas of our brains that control our memory, blood pressure, heart rate, hormone balance, breathing and stress levels, can be significantly influenced by essential oils that are able to reach the limbic system, bypassing the cerebral cortex. This is important in that once inhaled, they will affect both the physiological and psychological function of the body with positive results.

"Fragrance is one of man's greatest enjoyments, bringing back memories of past experiences and creating a feeling of security, grounding, and well-being. Dr. Joseph Ledoux, of New York Medical University, feels that this could be a significant breakthrough in releasing emotional trauma."

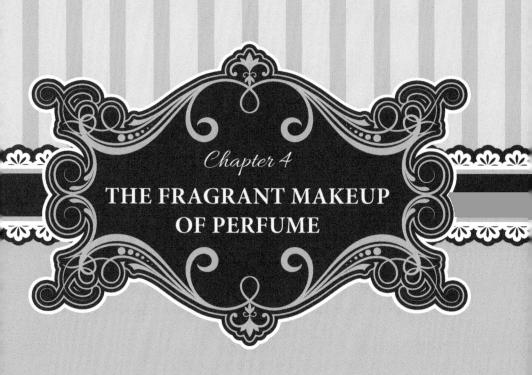

Chapter 4

THE FRAGRANT MAKEUP
OF PERFUME

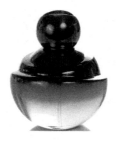

Happiness is perfume, you can't pour it on somebody else without getting a few drops on yourself.

– James Van Der Zee

The International Fragrance Association (IFRA) defines natural fragrances as "complex fragrance compounds made exclusively from natural aromatics." All of the ingredients used in natural fragrances are physically obtained from plants without altering their chemical structure. Aromatic components may include essential oils, absolutes, oleoresins, concretes, distillates, and fractions.

FRAGRANCE INGREDIENTS

In perfumery, various ingredients go into creating a perfume. Fragrances can be categorized into either chemical or natural perfumes based on the ingredients used to make them. Chemical components utilized in the composition of a fragrance may come from natural or synthetic means.

ESSENTIAL OILS

Essential oils and absolutes will be the building blocks of your perfume. These plant-based materials will provide fragrance, texture, and color to your product. Essential oils contain a complex amalgamation of natural compounds, which determine their fragrance and therapeutic properties. The chemical composition of an essential oil can be affected by its climatic conditions, pollutant exposure, extraction process and other factors that may influence its aroma.

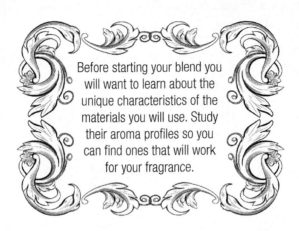

Before starting your blend you will want to learn about the unique characteristics of the materials you will use. Study their aroma profiles so you can find ones that will work for your fragrance.

The average essential oil contains around 100 to 300 components, along with thousands of other trace compounds that have yet to be identified by scientists. While attempts have been made to single out and synthetically duplicate identifiable components, nature far exceeds laboratory efforts and continues to remain mostly a mystery in their unique makeup. Essential oils will be covered in more detail in a later chapter.

AROMA CHEMICALS
Since these numerous factors can cause an essential oil's fragrance to alter from year to year, individual components in oil may be extracted to control the consistency of an aroma or to remove undesirable qualities. These are known as "aroma chemicals."

Aroma chemicals are sourced from isolates found in essential oils, chemically modified isolates, and the petrochemical industry. You may already be familiar with fragrant oils, aroma chemicals, and natural oils. In this book, our focus will be working only with essential oils in their natural state.

ABSOLUTES
Absolutes are concentrated aromatic oils extracted from plant material by solvent extraction. These are very similar to essential oils and are frequently used in perfumery because the aromatic compounds in absolutes did not undergo high temperatures during distillation. Examples of oils that are absolutes include rose otto and jasmine.

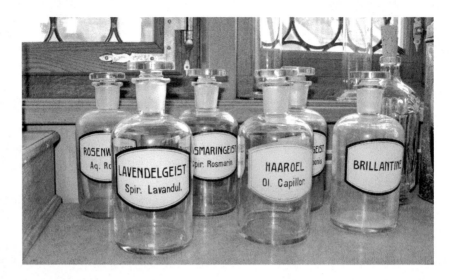

CARRIERS

There are several options to choose from when selecting a carrier agent to use with your custom-designed fragrance. Alcohols, oils, and waxes are all used to produce different types of products, and the one you choose will depend on the purpose of your blend and how you will want to apply it.

SO WHAT EXACTLY IS A CARRIER AGENT, ANYWAY?

A carrier agent is a substance or material that helps carry the scent of your fragrance. It serves three important functions: the carrier agent protects the wearer, lifts and carries the scent, and dilutes the essential oils in your blend. Most essential oils should not be applied directly to the skin, so diluting the oils in a carrier is the best way to place a protective barrier between you and the ingredients in your formula. Keep in mind that "less is more," especially for essential oils. Another benefit to using a carrier is to "lift" the scent so others can smell your perfume. This is why alcohol is such a popular choice in perfumes, because as it evaporates, it deposits the scent into the air around you. For a longer lasting fragrance, oils and wax hold the perfume against the body so that it can be absorbed into your skin. The strength and form of your perfume will determine which carrier agent is the right one for you.

ALCOHOL

Perfumer's alcohol is the most popular carrier agent for perfume. Angie Andriot, owner of Vetiver Aromatics, says, "Perfumer's Alcohol is the most popular carrier agent for perfume oils because of its method of application. The alcohol allows your perfume to be spritzed anywhere you would like to apply your fragrance. As the alcohol in the perfume evaporates, it carries the scent away from you and allows for a stronger presence" ("Perfumer's Alcohol," Vetiver Aromatics https://vetiveraromatics.com/products/perfumers-alcohol).

A perfumer's alcohol blend widely used in the professional perfume industry is SDA 40B. Pure grain alcohol, 200 proof, can also be made into all of your custom creations such as perfume, eau de parfum, eau de toilette, cologne, eau de cologne, after-bath spray and air freshener!

Most perfumes use alcohol as the preferred carrier agent. Because of its disinfectant properties, it will preserve the ingredients and give the blend a longer shelf life. You will want to make sure you choose the best alcohol available. Here are your options:

1. ***Perfumer's alcohol*** – This is the ideal choice, but can be very expensive and difficult to obtain. Special formulations are available online that are used by professionals and amateurs, which will help your formulas remain free from cloudiness. Keep in mind, though, perfumer's alcohol 40B contains ethanol (denatured), Isopropyl myristate, and Monopropylene glycol. These added ingredients to the denatured alcohol aid in absorption and act as a cosolvent to allow the oils to be solubilized and prevents evaporation in the alcohol carrier.
   Ethyl alcohol is available in two types: denatured and undenatured. Commercial perfumers use denatured alcohol. Handle with care as both are flammable and should be stored away from heat and light.

2. ***Everclear*** – This is pure grain alcohol, which can be purchased at most liquor stores.

3. ***Vodka*** – Be sure to use the highest proof you can find.
   Warning: *Do not use rubbing alcohol.*

If you are planning on reselling your products, you will need to check your government regulations regarding the usage and resell of alcohol. For US citizens, you will need a user permit from the Alcohol and Tobacco Tax and Trade Bureau. Visit the TTB permit website for more information at https://ttbonline.gov/permitsonline.

BEESWAX

Beeswax, an ancient and natural carrier, is ideal for creating a solid perfume, says Angie Andriot of Vetiver Aromatics. Her company offers cosmetic-grade beeswax that has been refined to purify and remove any residue from being in the honeycomb. With a natural soft yellow hue and hints of pleasant honey, it comes in beads that melt quickly in a double boiler. Beeswax is well known for its fixative properties, helping to anchor more volatile fragrance notes, and is perfect for those working within a natural perfumery palate. It is recommended to use unbleached natural beads or pellets. These will add a honey scent and beautiful consistency to your product.

CARRIER OILS

Carrier oils are mostly vegetable-based fatty oils used for diluting essential oils and as a method of application when applying essential oils to the body. You will need to have carrier oils on hand for creating solid perfumes and perfume oils.

Common carrier oils such as fractionated coconut and jojoba are easy to use when making body oils. These are favorite choices for many perfumers too, since they are odorless and have a nice light texture that is quickly absorbed into the skin. Another advantage to using a natural carrier oil is that they are much more subtle and do offer more "stay on" power. Fractionated coconut oil is colorless and less likely to stain clothing.

Jojoba oil is widely used in many skin and hair care products around the world and is a preferred carrier for many perfume oils because it closely resembles human sebum, a natural oil your skin and hair produces. It has a faint honey color with a slight nutty odor. Both jojoba oil and coconut oil have an indefinite shelf life.

JOJOBA OIL

Jojoba oil is bright and golden in color and is known as one of the best oils (actually a liquid wax) for hair and skin. Jojoba is suitable for all aromatherapy uses other than a full-body massage. And, because of the oil's antioxidants, it does not become rancid and can even prevent rancidity in other oils.

COCONUT OIL

Fractionated coconut oil seems to be the carrier oil of choice because of its vast use in aromatherapy and perfumery. While it is fractionated, no change has been made chemically. Rather, its molecular structure 'fraction' has been separated allowing it to remain liquid at room temperature—this makes it much more useful in creating perfume oils. Coconut oil is perfect as a moisturizer for the body and conditions brittle, dry or dull hair. Its light, easily absorbable texture gives skin a smooth satiny effect with virtually no scent of its own and an indefinite shelf life.

THE FRAGRANT MAKEUP OF PERFUME

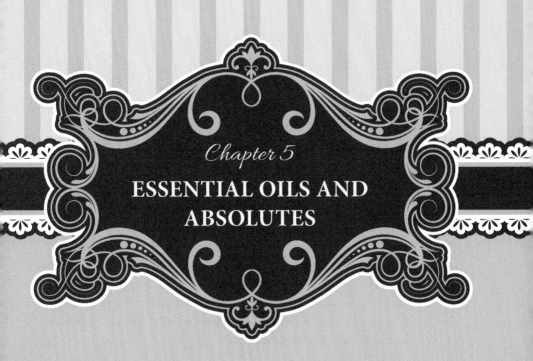

Chapter 5

ESSENTIAL OILS AND
ABSOLUTES

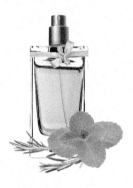

A perfume must be more mysterious than a copy of something in nature. When a man sees a woman, he shouldn't think of a rose; he should think of that woman.

– PERFUMER JEAN PAUL GUERLAIN ON THE PHILOSOPHY OF HIS GRANDFATHER JACQUES GUERLAIN

D id you know that it takes 60,000 rose blossoms to produce one ounce of rose oil? Have you ever given any thought to how much a rose petal weighs? Let's just say not very much, which is why it takes 2,300 pounds of rose petals to make a single pound of oil. Lavender, on the other hand, yields approximately seven pounds of oil from 220 pounds of dried flowers. Also, flowers must be picked by hand early in the morning before the sun rises and heats up, evaporating the essential oil within the petals. Hence, you can understand the variation in the pricing of various essential oils on the market.

A sandalwood tree must be thirty years old and over thirty feet tall before it can be cut down for distillation. Myrrh, frankincense, and benzoin oils are extracted from the gum resins of their respective trees. Citrus oils such as grapefruit, lime and lemon are extracted from the fruit's rind. Cinnamon essential oil comes from the bark and leaf of the tree while pine comes from the needles and twigs. With such a variety of essential oils and plant parts from which oils are extracted, there are several

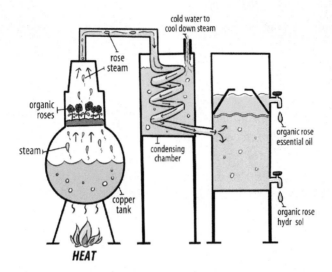

Diagram labels:
- cold water to cool down steam
- rose steam
- organic roses
- steam
- condensing chamber
- copper tank
- organic rose essential oil
- organic rose hydr sol

HEAT

methods used for extraction. The most common methods include steam distillation, solvent extraction, expression, enfleurage, and maceration.

STEAM DISTILLATION uses steam to extract the essential oils from the plant by suspending the plant material over water in a sealed container, which is then brought to a boil. The steam containing the volatile essential oil is run through a cooler, and once it condenses the liquid is collected. The essential oil appears as a thin layer on top of the fluid, as water and essential oils do not mix. The essential oil is separated from the water and is collected in a small vial while the water runs into a large vat.

SOLVENT EXTRACTION uses very little heat to preserve the oil which would otherwise be destroyed or altered during steam distillation. Fragile plant material such as jasmine, hyacinth, narcissus, or tuberose is dissolved in a liquid solvent of heptane, hexane, or methylene chloride as a suitable perfume solvent, which absorbs the smell, color, and wax of the plant. After removing the plant material, the solvent is boiled off under a vacuum to help separate the essential oil. Once the solvent evaporates, a substance called 'concrete' remains. The concrete is mixed with alcohol to aid in filtering the waxes, and distilling the alcohol away leaves an 'absolute.' The word 'absolute' appears on the label of some bottled essential oils, and because it may still contain 2-3 percent of the solvent, it is not considered pure essential oil.

Expression is how citrus oils are extracted. The essential oil from citrus fruits such as orange, lemon, lime and grapefruit is located in tiny sacs just beneath the surface of the rind. To extract the oil, it must be squeezed out or expressed from the peels and seeds by rolling the fruit over a conveyor containing short needles, which pierce the small oil pockets in the citrus fruit's rind. As the oil runs out, it is then collected and filtered.

*E*ssential oils are distilled from multiple parts of the plant including leaves, flowers, roots, seeds, bark, and resins, or expressed from the rinds of citrus fruits. It takes at least 50 pounds of plant material to make one pound of essential oil. For example, a pound of rosemary oil requires sixty-six pounds of herbs.

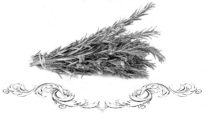

Enfleurage is an ancient method of extracting oils that is rarely used today because of its long, complicated and expensive process. Fragrant blooms were placed upon sheets of warm animal fat (or long layers of vegetable fat) to absorb the essential oil. As flowers were exhausted, they were replaced with fresh blossoms. This process was repeated until the sheet of fat was saturated with oil and finally separated with solvents leaving only the essential oil.

Maceration is a process in which plant material is gathered and chopped, and then added to either sunflower or olive oil. The mixture is stirred and placed in the sunlight for several days. This process transfers all of the soluble components from the plant material including its essential oil into the carrier oil, which is then carefully filtered. This process leaves a carrier oil infused with essential oil.

While there are several methods of extracting essential oils, steam distillation is the most common method. Other popular alternatives to traditional steam distillation include turbo distillation, hydro diffusion, and hypercritical carbon dioxide extraction.

TURBO DISTILLATION is a quick method in which plants are soaked in water, and steam is circulated and recycled through the plant mixture. This method is appropriate for essential oils that are extracted from coarse plant material such as bark, roots, and seeds.

HYDRO DIFFUSION is a steam distillation process in which steam is dispersed through the plant material from the top of the plant chamber, saturating the plants more evenly and taking less time than steam distillation. This method is considered less harsh than steam distillation with essential oils smelling much more like the original plant.

HYPERCRITICAL CARBON DIOXIDE (CO_2) EXTRACTION uses carbon dioxide under extremely high pressure to extract the essential oil. Plant materials are enclosed in a stainless steel tank where carbon dioxide is injected, and pressure builds. When the carbon dioxide turns into a liquid, it acts as a solvent for extracting the essential oils from the plants. Once the pressure is lessened, the carbon dioxide returns to a gaseous state, leaving no residues behind. Carbon dioxide extracted oils have a crisper aroma, smell more similar to the living plant and produce a higher yield from the plant material. This method provides a more potent oil with greater therapeutic benefits.

The recipes contained in this book are designed for essential oils, as better perfumes often come from a blend of essential oils. However, there is no reason you cannot use fragrance oils. In fact, some suggest starting with the much lower-cost fragrance oils until you understand the blending process. This will save you a lot of money until you discover which scent works for your skin, but be prepared to move onto pure essential oils for the best results.

WHAT IS THE DIFFERENCE BETWEEN A FRAGRANCE OIL AND AN ESSENTIAL OIL? HOW DO I KNOW WHICH ONE TO USE?

Essential oils are a natural byproduct derived from flowers and plants, whereas fragrance oils are most often a synthetic blend of ingredients diluted in a carrier oil. If you have been shopping online for oils to make perfume, you will notice a considerable difference in price between the two. You will find fragrance oils much cheaper. This is because it takes several hundreds of pounds of plant material to distil essential oils, which makes them more expensive.

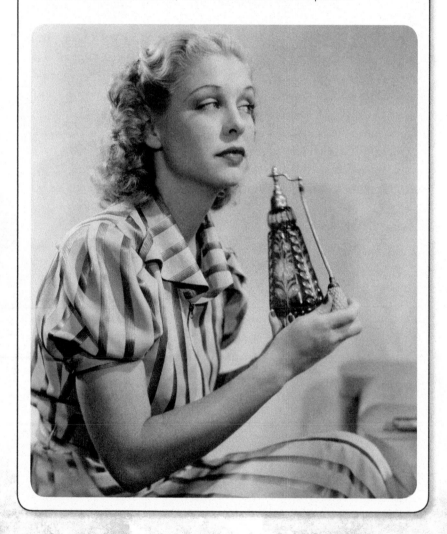

You will find some scents only available in fragrance oils such as banana, strawberry, mango, and sea and sand. Many people like the exotic and/or unique fragrances; however, they do not offer the natural health benefits you will find in pure essential oils derived from plants. Also, some people are allergic to fragrance oils and may suffer an allergic reaction.

Ultimately, the choice is yours. You will want to weigh the pros and cons of which oils to use, but if you want to create more advanced perfumes, use essential oils.

LIVING PLANT AND HEADSPACE TECHNOLOGY

In 1977, a gateway to a whole new realm of fragrance burst open. A paper about "Headspace Technology and Living Plants" by Dr. B. T. Mookherjee, R. W. Trenkle, and R. A. Wilson gave the perfume industry radical new insights into how essential oils from living plants differ from those taken from flowers cut just moments before.

For the experiment a glass flask called a Tenex trap was fixed securely around the head of the plant, encapsulating the flower in an airtight space, and steam was purged through it for several hours. The first comparison done was of living and cut blossoms from *Jasminum grandiflorum*, and the second from a yellow hybrid tea rose.

In comparisons the results were startling. In standard essential oil, benzyl acetate (one of the primary components of the scent of jasmine) makes up 40% of the oil. However, the volatiles collected from the living plant showed a massive increase to 60% of the oil.

The results from the yellow rose showed similar changes. This time there was a reduction in cis-3-hexenol from 20% in the living rose to just 5% in the oil from the cut bloom. This constituent has a very green note and is often synthetically added to give flavor to green tea, for instance. Quite literally the freshness of the aroma begins to die almost instantly.

Continuing the comparisons, Mookherjee tested lily of the valley, freesias, and *stephanotis*; in each case the findings were the same. The fragrance from the living plant was different from the cut one.

He then proceeded to investigate whether there were differences between flowers with different-colored blooms. The rose, of course, had to take precedence here. Most perfumers would seek to emulate the scent of the rose by trying to simulate a copy of *Rosa damascena*, a very ancient rose grown mainly in Bulgaria and considered to be the finest of all roses.

Studying blooms from five different-colored roses, however, showed the aroma profiles of various colored roses, in fact, vary considerably. Analyses were done on blooms from Red Chrysler Imperial, White JFK, Red/Yellow Double Delight, Purple Intrigue, and Otto of Rose Bulgarian. The primary constituent of the deep red Damascena is nerol-geranio and has a sweet rosy scent. The results of the test showed volatiles made up 30% of the Bulgarian Otto. In Purple Intrigue, it made just 2.6%. In the other roses, there was no presence at all.

By contrast, the Red Chrysler had high levels of citronellol, a much lighter floral rose-like fragrance and 3,5-Dimethoxy toluene, which is most usually only found in roses of Chinese origin. The headspace of each rose was entirely different from rose to rose, even having completely unique chemicals contained in each.

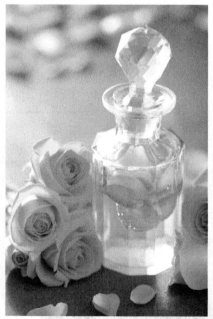

What, then, would the headspace show in plants that change their scents from night to day? On examination, honeysuckle showed a significant increase in the linalool in its nighttime profile. The levels rocket from 17% of the oil up to double the volume at 34%. Tuberose was more complicated; its limonene levels change from 8% to 14% at nightfall, but its methyl salicylate and alpha terpineol levels both drop radically. Its scent does not only increase; it dramatically alters.

Headspace and living technology has overhauled the way we use scent. Suddenly it is possible to create a myriad of new fragrances simply by varying the time of day they are taken and choosing whether they are gathered from living or dead plant matter.

COMMON AND BOTANICAL NAMES OF ESSENTIAL OILS

COMMON NAME	BOTANICAL NAME
Ajowan	Trachyspermum copticum
Angelica Root	Angelica archangelica
Anise	Pimpinella anisum
Balsam Fir	Abies balsams
Balsam, Copaiba	Copaifera officinalis
Balsam, Gurjun	Dipterocarpus turbinatus
Balsam, Peru	Myroxylon peruiferum
Basil	Ocimum basillicum
Bay Laurel	Laurus nobilis
Benzoin	Styrax benzoin
Bergamot	Citrus bergamia
Birch, Yellow	Betula alleghaniensis
Black Pepper	Piper nigrum
Blue Tansy	Tanacetum annum
Cajeput	Melaleuca leucadendra
Camphor	Cinnamomum camphora
Caraway Seed	Carum carvi
Cardamom	Elettaria cardamomum
Carrot Seed	Daucua carota
Cassia	Cinnamomum cassia
Cedar, Canadian Red	Thuja plicata
Cedar, Western Red	Thuja plicata
Cedar Leaf (Thuja)	Thuja occidentalis
Cedarwood	Cedrus atlantica
Chamomile, German	Matricaria recutita
Chamomile, Roman	Chamaemelum nobile
Cinnamon Bark	Cinnamomum verum
Cinnamon Leaf	Cinnamomum verum
Cistus Labdanum	Cistus ladanifer
Citronella	Cymbopogon nardus

COMMON NAME	BOTANICAL NAME
Clary Sage	*Salvia sclarea*
Clove Bud	*Syzygium aromaticum*
Coriander	*Coriandrum savitum L.*
Cumin	*Cuminum cyminum*
Cypress	*Cupressus sempervirens*
Cypress, Blue	*Callitris intratropica*
Davana	*Artemisia pallens*
Dill	*Anethum graveolens*
Douglas Fir	*Pseudotsuga menziesii*
Elemi	*Canarium luzonicum*
Eucalyptus	*Eucalyptus globulus*
Eucalyptus Citriodora	*Eucalyptus citriodora*
Eucalyptus Dives	*Eucalyptus dives*
Eucalyptus Polybractea	*Eucalyptus polybractea*
Eucalyptus Radiata	*Eucalyptus radiata*
Fennel	*Foeniculum vulgare*
Fir (Silver Fir or Fir Needle)	*Abies alba*
Fir Balsam (Canadian Balsam)	*Abies balsamea*
Fir (White or Idaho Balsam)	*Abies grandis*
Fleabane	*Erigeron annuus*
Frankincense (Olibanum)	*Boswellia carterii*
Galbanum	*Ferula gummosa*
Garlic	*Allium sativum*
Geranium	*Pelargonium graveolens*
Ginger	*Zingiber officinale*
Goldenrod	*Solidago canadensis*
Grapefruit	*Citrus x paradisi*
Helichrysum	*Helichrysum italicum*
Helichrysum	*Helichrysum odoratissimum*
Ho Wood	*Cinnamomum camphora*
Hyssop	*Hyssopus officinalis*
Idaho Tansy	*Tanacetum vulgare*
Inula	*Inula graveolens*
Jasmine	*Jasminum officinale*
Juniper	*Juniperus osteosperma or J. scoluporum*
Lavandin	*Lavandula x hybrida*
Lavender	*Lavandula angustifolia, CT Linalool*

COMMON NAME	BOTANICAL NAME
Lemon	*Citrus limon*
Lemongrass	*Cymbopogon flexuous*
Lime	*Citrus aurantifolia*
Linaloe Berry	*Bursera delpechian*
Mandarin	*Citrus reticulate*
May Chang	*Litsea cubeba*
Melaleuca (Tea Tree)	*Melaleuca alternifolia*
Melissa (Lemon Balm)	*Melissa officinalis*
Mugwort (Wormwood)	*Artemisia vulgaris*
Myrrh	*Commiphora myrrha*
Myrtle	*Myrtus communis*
Neroli (Orange Blossom)	*Citrus aurantium bigaradia*
Niaouli	*Melaleuca quinquenervia*
Nutmeg	*Myristica fragrans*
Oakmoss (Green moss or Lichen)	*Evernia prunastri*
Onycha (Benzoin)	*Styrax benzoin*
Orange, Blood	*Citrus sinensis*
Orange, Sweet	*Citrus sinensis*
Oregano	*Origanum vulgare, CT Carvacrol*
Palmarosa	*Cymbopogon martinii*
Palo Santo (Holy Wood)	*Bursera graveolens*
Parsley Seed	*Petroselinum sativum*
Patchouli	*Pogostemon cablin*
Peppermint	*Mentha piperita*
Petitgrain	*Citrus aurantium*
Pimento Leaf	*Pimenta dioica*
Pine, Scotch	*Pinus sylvestris*
Plai	*Zingiber cassumunar*
Ravensara	*Ravensara aromatica*
Ravintsara	*Cinnamomum camphora*
Rosalina	*Melaleuca ericifolia*
Rose Otto, Bulgarian	*Rosa damascena*
Rosemary Cineol	*Rosemarinus officinalis, CT 1,8 Cineole*
Rosemary Verbenon	*Rosemarinus officinalis, CT Verbenone*
Rosewood	*Aniba rosaeodora*
Sage	*Salvia officinalis*
Sandalwood	*Santalum album*

COMMON NAME	BOTANICAL NAME
Savory, Wild	*Satureja montana*
Spearmint	*Mentha spicata, CT Carvone*
Spikenard	*Nardostachys jatamansi*
Spruce, Black	*Picea mariana*
Spruce, Blue (Hemlock)	*Tsuga canadensis*
Spruce, White	*Picea glauca*
Tagetes	*Tagetes minuta*
Tamanu	*Catophyllum inophylllum*
Tangerine	*Citrus nobilis*
Tansy, Blue	*Tanacetum annum*
Tansy, Idaho	*Tanacetum vulgare*
Tarragon	*Artemisia dracunculus*
Thyme	*Thymus vulgaris, CT Thymol*
Thyme Linalol	*Thymus vulgaris, CT Linalool*
Tsuga (Hemlock)	*Tsuga canadensis*
Turmeric	*Curcuma longa*
Valerian	*Valeriana officinalis*
Vanilla Oleoresin	*Vanilla planifolia*
Verbena, Lemon	*Lippia citriodora*
Verbena, Rosemary	*Rosmarinus officinalis, CT Verbenone*
Vetiver	*Vetiveria zizanoides*
White Lotus	*Nymphaea lotus*
Winter Savory	*Satureja montana*
Wintergreen	*Gaultheria procumbens*
Wormwood (Mugwort)	*Artemisia vulgaris*
Yarrow	*Achillea millefolium*
Ylang Ylang	*Cananga odorata*

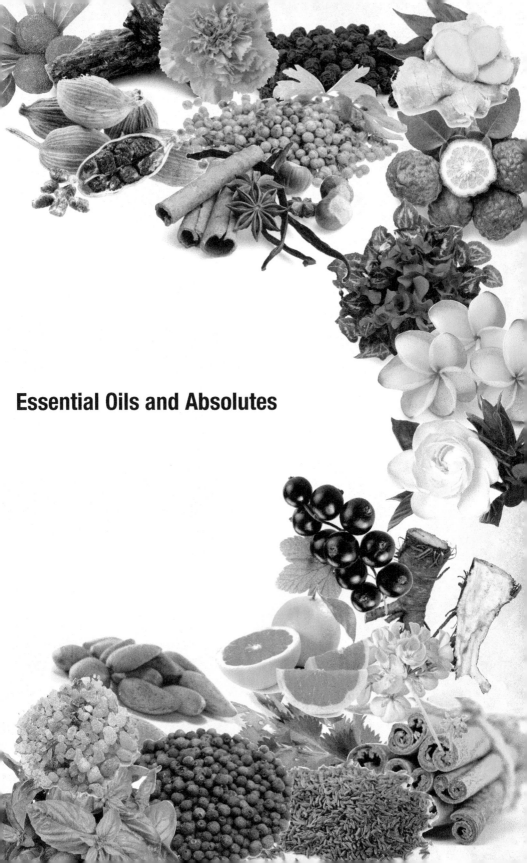

Essential Oils and Absolutes

ALLSPICE

Native to Central America, the Caribbean, and Mexico, Allspice is now cultivated in many warm climates. The Jamaican pepper, myrtle pepper or new spice uses the dried fruit of the evergreen *Pimenta doica* plant. Combining the flavors of cinnamon, nutmeg and clove, it has a sharp but spicy heart note. It heats up chypre blends in particular and contains the chemical constituent caryophyllene alcohol, which has a green, floral edge.

Found in:

Bois d'hiver and *Sabotage* - Ayala Moriel

Frankincense and *Allspice* - Molton Browns

Allure Homme - Chanel

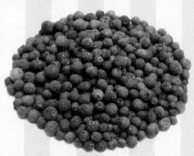

AMBER

Amber is a fossilized resin secreted by the now extinct Pinus succinifera tree. The resin is blended with sunflower and jojoba carrier oils as well as spikenard, vetiver, myrrh and frankincense essential oils to allow it to release the warm, sweet, woody note. Known by such romantic titles as Tigers Soul, Petrified Light, and Hardened Honey, this oil is a combination of labdanum, benzoin, and vanilla and is found extensively in oriental and chypre blends.

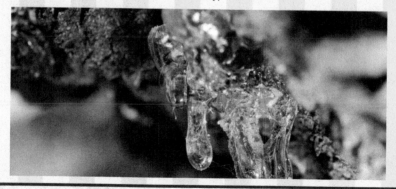

AMBRETTE SEED

The exotic and lofty Musk Mallow is the source of this absolute, which is usually extracted by CO_2.

Its animalistic, musky and almost metallic fragrance for many years was used in perfume as an alternative plant-derived fixative to musk. Its high price tag has prompted the creation of synthetic alternatives that are now more often used in fragrance creation.

It has a dry, sultry note and a very masculine dimension to the aphrodisiac qualities that lend to oriental and floral accords.

Found in:

Homme Intense - Dior

Beauty - Calvin Klein

Rose The One - Dolce & Gabanna

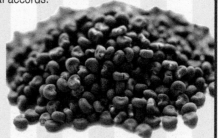

ANGELICA

A tall, statuesque and willowy plant from the Umbelliferae family, angelica has stalks that are sweet and edible. Previously native to Europe and Siberia, angelica now grows freely across the globe, especially on well-watered riverbanks. It flowers between June and August, and both roots and seeds are used to extract the essential oil by steam distillation. In fact, the oil can refer to any one of 60 species from which it can be extracted. It is the roots that give the distinctive flavor to gin.

Its aromatic, green, spicy, peppery note has a musky animal edge to it.

Found in:

Angelique Noire - Guerlain

Angelique sous la pluie - Frédéric Malle

Versace Man - Versace

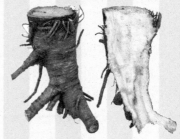

ANISE

This green, spicy aromatic oil should not be confused with the similarly named Star Anise. This oil is taken from the Umbelliferae plant native to Asia and gives the distinctive licorice, aniseed aroma.

Extracted from the leaves by steam distillation, anise is often used to warm woody chypre blends.

The plant aids with digestion and is highly fragranced and flavorsome. For this reason, the Romans used it in a cake called Mustaceum that they would serve at special occasions. It is believed this could be the origins of wedding cake.

Found in:

007 Ocean Royale - James Bond

Apparition Homme Intense - Ungaro

Armani Code - Armani

BALSAM OF PERU

You will also see this listed as Tolu Balsam, a large, aggressive tree that is extremely invasive and has the capacity to wipe out other indigenous species entirely. The term Peru Balsam is a misnomer as initially it was found along the coast of El Salvador.

The largest producers now of this sweet, fresh earthy scented oil are France and Central America.

The lush, warm, opulent floral note lends itself well to heavy, warm winter fragrances.

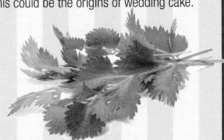

Found in:

Vol de Nuit Shalimar Eau de Cologne - Guerlain

Youth Dew - Estée Lauder

Elixir de Merveilles - Hermes

BASIL

This herbaceous, green and refreshing plant originally came from India and found its way to Europe along the spice routes. It became a vital part of both Mediterranean and Thai cooking.

All nations agree that basil is a regal plant. It takes its name from the Greek word meaning "kingly" or "royal."

In Romania, it has romantic undertones as a prospective groom accepts a sprig of basil from his fiancée when he becomes engaged.

The aromatic note of basil is bright, abrasive and peppery; it adds a touch of sunshine in a blend, especially for floral and citrus fragrances.

Found in:

Green Water - Jacques Faith

Armani Eau Pour Hommes - Armani

Eau Sauvage - Dior

Aquascutum - London

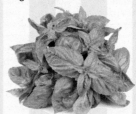

BAYBERRY

Taken from a different plant than the bay leaf, this one is extracted from Myrica cerifera. It was extensively used in nineteenth century colonial American medicine and grows expansively in America and Canada. In the early 1800s, bayberry candles were burnt for their light and clear scent.

It has a woody, balsam fragrance with spicy undertones of nutmeg and ginger.

This is the bay that is commonly called Bay Rum.

Found in:

L'humaniste - Frapin

Happy Woman - E D May

Baudelaire - Byredo Parfum

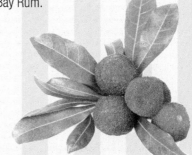

BENZOIN

This resin is taken from the Styrax benzoin tree. A stubby tree with gray bark, the finest of this oil is collected from the areas of Laos from the Styrax tonkinensis.

Its delicious vanilla scent makes a wonderful fixative and so has historically been connected with incense. The gorgeous gum of benzoin has a woody and spicy note.

Found in:

Prada Candy - Prada

Cinema - Yves Saint Laurent

Velvet Wood - Dolce & Gabbana

BERGAMOT

Originating from the town of Bergamo in Southern Italy, a bergamot is a pear-shaped green orange; a hybrid between a Seville orange and a grapefruit.

Although now it can also be propagated along the Ivory Coast, Argentina and Brazil, these fruits are considered to be inferior containing less fructose than those grown in Italy.

The bergamot is inedible although it is sometimes used as flavoring in, for instance, Earl Grey tea. On the whole, though, it is created purely for perfumery purposes. Its sweet, fruity, and mildly spicy note is quintessential to chypres and fougère fragrances.

Found in:

Attraction Summer - Lancôme

Marco Polo Pure Morning Woman - Marco Polo

212 Men Splash - Carolina Herrera

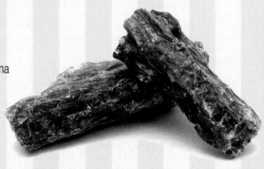

BITTER ALMOND

Historically, this oil was taken from the kernels of bitter almond tree—*Prunus dulcis var amara* as opposed to *Prunus dulcis var amygdalus*, which refers to the sweet almonds we enjoy eating). However, in the nineteenth century, this oil began to be synthetically made because of the high levels of cyanide in the oil.

Today, the oil is synthetically created from the kernels of peach, apricot, cherry or plum. You will see it labeled as FFPA, which means Free From Prussic Acid, the old name for hydrocyanic acid.

Bitter almond is the strongest version of an almond fragrance you will ascertain.

Found in:

Omnia - Bvlgari

Hypnotic Poison - Dior

Mon Precieux Nectar - Guerlain

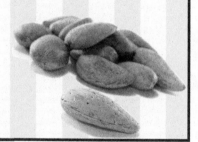

BITTER ORANGE

This zesty and refreshing note blends the sweetness of oranges with the slight bitterness of grapefruit. Oils in the citrus family are said to have a hesperedic note, a sweet and uplifting feel to them. As one would imagine, this oil is the bitter end of the group.

The oil is expressed from the outer peel of the fruit of the same tree from which petitgrain (leaves) and neroli (orange blossom) are obtained. Originally this tree was only found in the Far East but now is produced extensively across the Mediterranean.

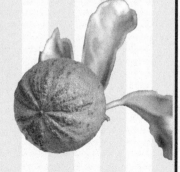

Found in:

Aqua Allegoria Mandarine Basilic - Guerlain

House of Matriarch - Christi Meshell

Citrico - Comme des Garcons

BLACK CURRANT BUD

This dark green absolute is solvent extracted mainly from bushes grown in Burgundy, France. Around 30 tons of flowers are harvested from three different types of black currant in the season between December and February. Its lush, spicy, fruitiness is topped with slightly acidic nuances of green tea. It is one of those scents that is entirely impossible to confuse with anything else, and reminiscent of childhood drinks from the old country!

There is a synthetic version which is called cassis. The natural compadré has a greener and lighter note to it.

Found in:

Lalique - Amethyst

Chamade - Guerlain

Be Delicious - DKNY

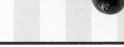

BLACK PEPPER

One of man's oldest spices, black pepper is extracted by steam distillation from the flowering, dried fruit of the bush native to South India. Historically known as *Black Gold*, it is the world's most traded spice. Nowadays the largest producer is Vietnam.

Its hot and bracing aura lends bright top accents to blends. Black pepper's spicy aromatic note warms them and brings cheerfulness.

Found in:

Notorious - Ralph Lauren

Omnia - Bvlgari

Sensuous - Estee Lauder

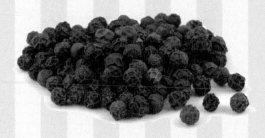

BOIS DE ROSE (ROSEWOOD)

Native to Brazil, rosewood is now a threatened species due to the extensive deforestation to create the oil, and synthetic versions are mainly used. Good practice is the use of the name "Bois de Rose" in order to avoid confusion with the wood that actually does come from roses!

The beautifully striated wood of the tree can run from brick red in color to a dark, almost violet shade. Having the most remarkable resonance, it has long been revered for its affinity to guitar and lute making.

It has a deliciously woody, mossy note with a light rosy accent, making it popular in both men's and women's fragrances.

Found in:

Rose Wood/Blackcurrant/Cyclamen - Korres

Eternity for Men - Calvin Klein

Lovely - Sarah Jessica Parker

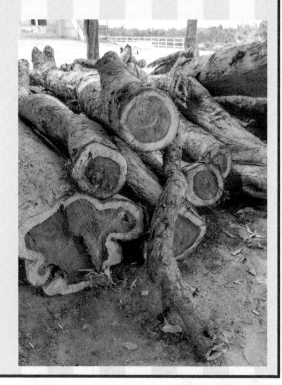

CARDAMOM

This intensely sweet, spicy note is steam distilled from green cardamom pods. The plant itself is a member of the ginger family. Cardamom is one of the most expensive spices in the world, rating only third after saffron and vanilla. It has a quintessentially Eastern feel to it.

For many generations in Egypt, the tradition was to chew cardamom to sweeten one's breath. In perfumery, it sweetens oriental blends and makes a sweet heart note in chypres.

Found in:

Saffron Amber Cardamom - Korres

Declaration - Cartier

Mabon - Fleurage Perfume Atelier

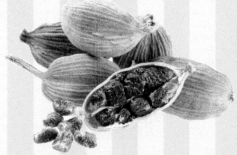

CARNATION

This is an absolute rather than an essential oil and is made only in France. It has a deep, lovely floral spiciness that is reminiscent of pepper and cloves. It is commonly used in fragrances to deepen floral notes.

In its own right it is seen as a very old-fashioned scent now (Lazell Pink Carnation dates back to 1897) and so is not used extensively alone but makes a valuable contribution to oriental blends.

Found in:

Pink Carnation - Lazell

Blue Carnation - Roger Gallet

Carnation - Comme des Garçons

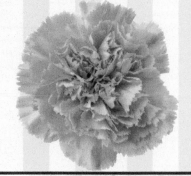

CARAWAY

The seeds of the tall plant from the Umbelliferae plant are steam distilled to produce essential oil. Again, we have a venerable and aged member of the fragrance groups, having been one of the first spices recorded in history.

The sweet, aniseed flavor and excellent digestive properties have made caraway a vital part of cuisines across the globe. The favorite Easter Simnel Cake is made almost exclusively from marzipan and caraway seeds. Traditionally, nuns who had taken sacred orders and were allowed to visit their families only once a year spent many hours creating their culinary masterpiece with eleven balls of marzipan (for the disciples of Jesus, excluding Judas) to present to their mothers on Mothering Sunday. In England, caraway is the quintessential taste of Easter.

The warm spiciness of the anise scent is found in all fragrance blends from orientals and fougères right through to florals and citrus blends.

Found in:

Cypress - Yves Saint Laurent

Magnifique - Lancôme

Le Male - Jean Paul Gaultier

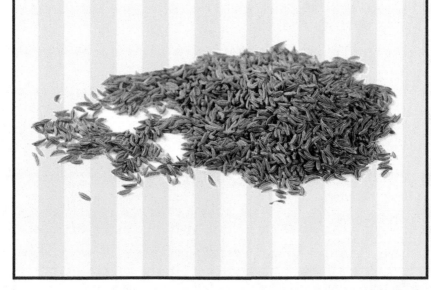

CASSIE

This subtle and intimate scent comes from the acacia tree. The extract is a solvent extracted absolute rather than an essential oil. It has a heady innocence to it with nuances of almonds to its fragrance. Often confused with mimosa, cassie has a dark richness similar to that of violet leaf and adds refinement to chypre fragrance blends.

Found in:

Une Fleur de Cassie - Frederic Malle

Après L'Ondée - Guerlain

Private Collection - Estée Lauder

CEDARWOOD

Austere and somber cedar is mostly found growing in the Himalayas and the Mediterranean. The essential oil is distilled from the leaves and sometimes branches and twigs of the tree.

It is a very ancient component that was used by the Egyptians in their embalming process. Since medieval times, its astringent scent has been used to care for garments by repelling moths.

The woody dryness of the oil makes a fantastic support to more cheerful notes and balances blends beautifully. This is one oil that exists in most perfumery blends, and is a very well used note.

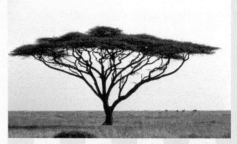

Found in:

Cedre - Serge Lutens

Gold for Woman - Amouage

Joy of Pink - Lacoste

CINNAMON/CASSIA

The inner bark of the cinnamon tree has been used since ancient times not only for its fragrance and flavor but also for its aphrodisiac reputation. The origins of this sharp, spicy ingredient trace back to Egypt 2000 BC, but it seems likely that it goes back even earlier to China.

Cassia, known as a cheaper cinnamon, is a tree having a similar scent and properties.

Found in:

Heart and Soul - LR

Sheherazade - Jean Desprez

Marc Jacobs Amber Perfume - Marc Jacobs

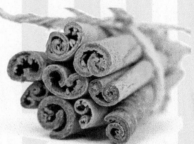

CORIANDER

Coriander essential oil is distilled from the seeds and the leaves of the cilantro plant. It has a woody, resinous clay-like scent that comes from the seeds, and the leaves give it a sharp, fresh, almost citrus-like herbaceous note.

It is a very ancient smell. The ancient Egyptians used to add the herb to wine and called the drink "the secret of happiness." Later archaeologists discovered coriander seeds in the tomb of Tutankhamen.

Found in:

Coriandre Perfume - Jean Couturier

Coriander Perfume - D.S. & Durga

Silver Shadow - Davidoff

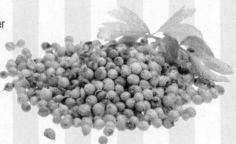

COSTUS

This strange, bodily scented oil is steam distilled from the root of the flower that is the symbol of Nigeria. The family it comes from is known as the Spiral Ginger, and has an intimate and comforting animalistic note. Some describe it like a wet dog, others say it smells like a newborn baby's head as it ages. However, it gains a far sweeter, rosier floral note.

Found in:

Solo Loewe - Loewe

Notes - Robert Piguet

A Taste of Heaven - Killian

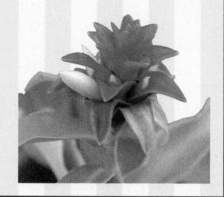

CYCLAMEN

This family has many species, and many of the flowers of these plants have little or no fragrance. This essential oil has a light, clean and almost mysterious air to it. It leaves a very slightly green edge to it. There is also an absolute made from cyclamen, but it is the essential oil that is mainly used.

Found in:

Vert d'Eau - Les Nereides

Insense Ultramarine Blue Sky - Givenchy

Curious - Brittany Spears

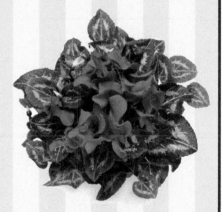

ELEMI

Extracted by steam distillation from the resin of the Canarium luzonicum tree, elemi has been used in medicine since the beginning of civilization. The ancient Egyptians employed elemi as a part of their embalming process; it is also mentioned in the ancient herbal writings of Pliny dating back to the first century AD. Today, it is predominately found growing in the Philippines.

This is a fresh and almost citrus scent having a close proximity to that of frankincense. It is often found in citrus and chypres blends.

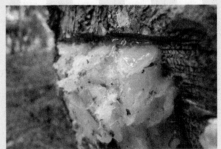

Found in:

L'instant de Guerlain pour homme - Guerlain

L'eau de Parfum Elemis - Elemis

L'heure mysterieuse - Cartier XII

EUGENOL

This extract can be taken from many sources such as nutmeg, clove, and vanilla, and is an active ingredient with anesthetic qualities. In perfumery, this yellow liquid brings a clearly clove-like scent. However, eugenol, when compared to oil of cloves, is more refined, less woody and has a muskier, more green note to perceive. Eugenol is often found as a delicious heart note of fougères creations.

Found in:

Opium - Yves Saint Laurent

Parfum Sacré - Caron

Chanel No. 5 - Chanel

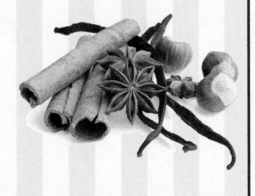

FRANGIPANI

Frangipani is an absolute obtained by solvent extraction from the plumeria flower. You may recognize these from flowers used in Polynesian leis. Traditionally, the women wore these flowers as a romantic signaling system to would-be advances. A flower worn over their left ear denoted they were looking for a suitor, and over the right gave a coy message they were already spoken for.

Frangipani is an exotic, heady and deeply sensual scent. The plant itself is far more fragrant at night in order to attract the Sphinx moth to pollinate it. It is considered a very seductive note found in chypre oriental and floral creations, which of course are designed as beguiling evening time wear.

Found in:

Frangipani - Ormonde Jayne

Beige - Chanel

Tocca - Stella

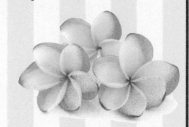

FRANKINCENSE

The Bible's most famous essential oil is distilled from the tears of resin, which form under the bark of the boswellia tree. The hard gum can only be harvested twice a year, once in the spring and once in the autumn, and takes two weeks to obtain sufficiently from the tree. Used extensively as incense, frankincense carries ritualistic significance throughout most of the world's religions. For many Eastern religions, it is used largely due to its ability to slow down the breath, making it perfect for bringing about a meditative state. The heady, almost antiseptic fragrance gives a vibrant and sharp resinous base note, especially to aromatic and woody blends.

Found in:

Messe de Minuit - Etro

Parfum Sacré - Caron

Gold - Amouge

FREESIA

Although the freesia does yield an essential oil, this is a synthetic fragrance laden with linalools, with a hint of jasmine to create a "super-fragrance." It is a refreshing, peppery, green fragrance rarely used alone. Freesia is predominately used as a modifier in blends.

Found in:

Musc & Freesia - E Coudray

Sheer Freesia - Oscar De La Renta

Wonderstruck Enchanted - Taylor Swift

GALBANUM

The unguent essential oil, which is distilled from the galbanum tears of resin, has an immediate shock of a mix of green pepper blended with hyacinth. When it dries down, though, it has a woody, earthy, sweet and sultry tone to it. This a very ancient component believed to be affiliated with Osiris, the ancient Egyptian god of the underworld. In the book of Exodus, the scriptures describe how the Lord told Moses to collect galbanum, which would later become one of the key components to make up the sacred incense of Solomon's Temple.

Found in:

Miss Dior - Dior

Chanel 19 - Chanel

Armani - Georgio Armani

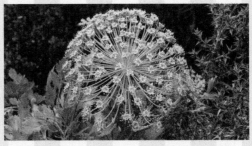

GARDENIA

Symbolic of love, this beautiful white flower has had many attempts to create an essential oil, but with no success. All essences of gardenia are synthetic, predominately made from blends of other flowers such as jasmine.

It is deliciously silky and floral. Gardenia perfume is so heady you feel as if you are drifting right through the top of your head!

Found in:

Gardenia - Chanel

Gardenia - Marc Jacobs

Gardenia - Annick Goutal

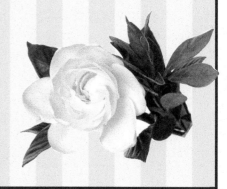

GERANIUM

Often confused with rose oil, geranium has a less powdery note and a more noticeably lemony scent to it. Taken from the flowers of this popular plant grown right across the globe, geranium can also be found in the form of geranium bourbon, which is the finest of all geraniums. Typically, the essential oil is used in perfumery, but there is also an olive-colored absolute that is often used in chypres and fougères.

Found in:

Geranium pour Monsieur d'Éditions - Frédéric Malle

Jeux de peau de parfum - Serge Lutens

Lola - Marc Jacobs

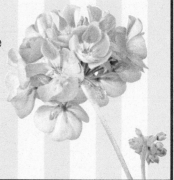

GINGER

Instantly recognizable in gingerbread, it is bright, sharp and warm. In fact, there are over 1,000 species of ginger with the whole plant being used to make essential oil. This warm, sweet, spicy note is an invaluable heart note in chypre fragrances and often adds to the sweetness of florals.

Found in:

Crystal Noir - Versace

Classique - Jean Paul Gautier

Rococo for Men - Joop

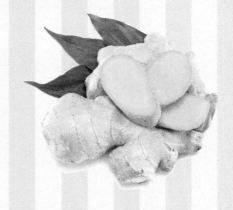

GRAPEFRUIT

The bright, sharp, lovely, slightly bitter fragrance comes from a relatively new fruit. Whereas almost other citruses came from the Old World, grapefruits were introduced from the Caribbean in the eighteenth century, and it seems likely were a hybrid of a pomelo and an orange. Now Florida is the largest producer, contributing a massive 1/3 of the world's grapefruits.

This is a succulent sour hesperedic note alongside all those other sweeter citruses.

Found in:

Pink Grapefruit - Floris

Gucci - Gucci Sport

1 Million for Men - Paco Rabanne

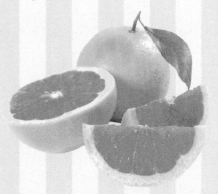

HELIOTROPE

A beautiful hedgerow shrub with bright purple flowers, it is a member of the borage family. Heliotrope's scent vacillates between marzipan and cherry pie, making it homely and inviting in blends. It is not possible to capture the fragrance in an essential oil, so both a maceration and an effleurage are created from the flower. In perfumery, though, a synthetic rendition usually utilizes the component heliotropin, a powdery vanilla fragranced constituent with the aroma of Italian meringue.

Found in:

Heliotrope Blanc for Women - L.T. Piver

Heliotrope Olivier for Women - Durbano

Cerruti Si Homme - Cerruti

HONEYSUCKLE

Known as the narcotic embrace of summer evenings, honeysuckle takes its name from its delicious nectar, which is, in truth, used to suckle children in some cultures. The scent is a heady, intoxicating aroma that is very difficult to blend with other notes. Those who do it with success are the works of very talented fragrance noses.

In many ways, it is similar to jasmine, but where jasmine is sultry and in some respects a little brooding, honeysuckle is fun, light-hearted and very much a "let's grab life while we can" type of vibration.

Found in:

Green Tea - Elizabeth Arden

Burberry Brit - Burberry

Fahrenheit - Dior

HYACINTH

As a bright, oily green floral note, the hyacinth scent has tremendous depth to it. There are three main colors of the bloom: pink, blue and white. As each flower blooms, the scent pervades stronger and stronger. Interestingly, each color has a discernibly different scent.

Due to the fragility of the flower, which does not lend itself well to distillation, hyacinth comes as a solvent extracted absolute.

Found in:

Bluebell (Woodland Hyacinth) - Penhaligon

Hyacinth Perfume - Yardley London

Ombre de Hyacinth - Tom Ford's Private Blend

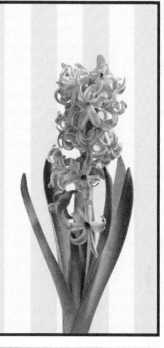

JASMINE

Where rose is the Queen of Flowers, jasmine is King. Fiercely expensive, 8,000 petals must be used to obtain just one milliliter of oil. Jasmine is an absolute obtained by solvent extraction. There are two types of jasmine used in perfumery: Jasminum grandiflorum and sambac. Both carry an almost trancelike headiness to their fragrance, which carries a very long way in nature. There are also synthesizations of the scent which tend to have a lighter, more airy feel to them.

Found in:

Australian Wild Jasmine for Women - Lucy B

Jasmine Noir Bluebeards Revenge - Bvlgari

Cool Water - Davidoff

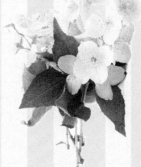

JONQUIL

Part of the narcissus family, the jonquil absolute is one of the most expensive perfume ingredients you can buy. It is so heady that undiluted members of this flower family can cause hallucinations. It is a changeable note and alters a great deal in drydown. In the first instance, it is deep, sweet and earthy with an almost animal-like quality. Jonquil has a long life, taking around three hours to reach the end of its change when it becomes powdery and honeyed. Used incorrectly, this can be a very cloying note.

Jonquil plays an integral part in perfumery and can be seen to be one of the predominant ingredients in Roman Perfumery. It is used, for obvious reasons, mainly in very expensive recipes, but this heady floral note is found in many French recipes.

Found in:

Ambre Cabochard - Parfums Gres

Pour Homme - Paco Rabanne

Declaration - Cartier

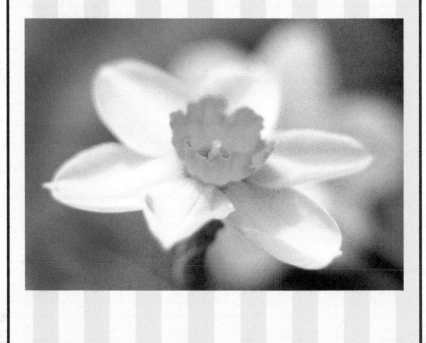

JUNIPER

The airy gin-like scent is captured by steam distillation from juniper berries. Man has a long relationship with the juniper tree; evidence shows that prehistoric man lived in close proximity to the juniper forests that furnished food, shelter, and fuel.

It is a source of debate as to just how many species of juniper there are; there are perhaps 52 to 67 depending on how the plants are classified. Currently, the groups include both needle-like leaves and scale leaves. This is a sharp, bitter aromatic note.

Found in:

Avalon Juniper - Pacifica

Juniper Sling - Penhaligon

Lacoste Elegance - Lacoste

LABDANUM

This is an oil that smells nothing like you would expect from the plant. Also known as Cistus ladanifer, labdanum is distilled from resins obtained from the rock rose flower. This intensely powerful and leathery scent is important to chypre perfumes. It also lends a nuance of an ambery note to orientals. Historically, it was collected from the beard of goats that had grazed on the mountains where it grew. Today, however, it is swept from the stems with a special broom.

Found in:

Omnia - Bvlgari

Oud Fleur - Tom Ford

Lavande - L'Occitane

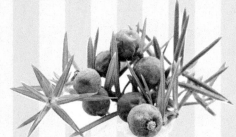

LAVANDIN

Lavandin is a hybrid of two lavender species that gives a very refreshing aromatic top-middle note to blends. English lavender was crossed with Spike lavender, which has a high camphorous content. It is considered a more hardy plant than lavender, being less susceptible to disease, which makes it an excellent alternative for the perfume industry. This more pungent, sharp tone is the clear differentiator between Lavender and Lavandin.

Found in:

Antidote - Viktor & Rolf

Lavandula - Penhaligons

Polo - Ralph Lauren

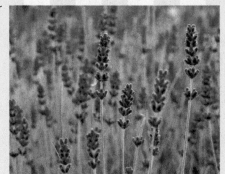

LAVENDER

A very ancient plant, its name lavender comes from the Latin laver, meaning "to wash." Indeed, it was the principle part of the Roman bathing regime. It has a sharp but sweet floral scent and tends to work very well in herbaceous blends. All fougères perfumes have lavender as their top note and oakmoss as their base.

Predominately essential oil is used, distilled from the flower heads and stalks, but it is also possible to obtain a thick, green absolute. This sweeter, more sugary fragrance is more soothing and woody than the essential oil.

Found in:

Lavender - Caswell Massey

Essence Lavender - Donna Karan

Encens de Lavande - Serge Lutens

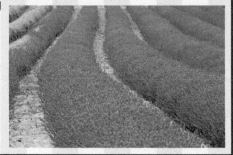

LEMONGRASS

With its sharp, zingy lemony-ginger scent, it has become well recognized in Eastern cookery. Some consider it pungent in how sharp and fresh it is.

Lemongrass is an aromatic hesperedic note that is often the bright top in chypre blends.

Found in:

Lemongrass e Cassis - Borsari

Eton College - Taylor of Old Bond Street

Pleasures Exotic - Estée Lauder

LEMON

Most are familiar with the sweet, yet sour fragrance of lemon. It brings a cheerful and vibrant feel to a blend. The oil obtained by the process of expression from the peel is perhaps a more astringent scent than the fruit itself. Lemon is the most acidic of hesperedic notes.

Found in:

Grass - Marc Jacobs

Plum - Mary Greenwell

Guilty Pour Homme - Gucci

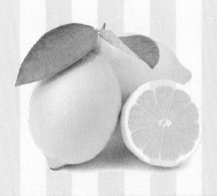

LILAC

It is a little-known fact that the lilac tree is part of the olive family and was brought to Vienna over 400 years ago from the Balkan Peninsula. Lilac flowers will only spring from old wood and so a lilac bush should rarely be pruned.

The ancient Celts believed the heady floral fragrance of lilac could transport a person to the land of fairies and magical beings. Its blend of honeyed nectar with memories of jasmine is believed in herbal medicine to restore joy and heal old memories.

Found in:

Lilac - Demeter

Floratta in Lilac for Women - O Boticario

Lilac - Gabels

LILY

There are oils from a number of different plants containing the name lily (water lily, lily of the valley, etc.) but this is obtained by distillation from the petals of the lilium family—those you would recognize from the garden with very long stems and large flower heads.

The perfume has a spicy but waxy note and is very sweetly floral. As it begins to dry down, it takes on a more salty brine nuance.

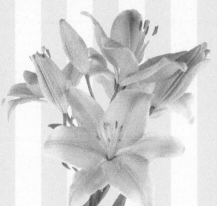

Found in:

Oscar Pink Lily - Oscar De La Renta

Lily Hearts - Femenino

Eternity for Men - Calvin Klein

LILY OF THE VALLEY

The beautiful flower of May is the pure essence of woodland spring. It has a bright, strong green floral note, but also encapsulates the headiness of jasmine; it is a very sweet scent.

Over time, its long waxy leaves and tiny white bells have come to symbolize purity, tenderness, and innocence, which seems slightly odd considering it is a highly poisonous plant.

Found in:

Lily of the Valley - Floris

Diorissimo - Dior

Opus 1870 - Penhaligans

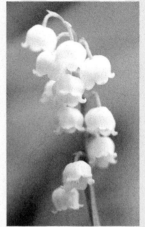

LIME

This green citrus fruit originally from Persia is sharper and more sour than a lemon. In the nineteenth century, sailors were prescribed a daily dose of lemon to prevent scurvy, which later limes were used because of the erroneous supposition they had a higher content of vitamin C. The oil, which is expressed from the peel, is usually combined with lemon to provide a sharp hesperedic top note to blends.

Found in:

Nina Gold Edition - Nina Ricci

Sweet Delicious Tart Key Lime - DKNY

Aromatic Lime - Montale

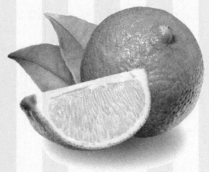

MACE/NUTMEG

Mace is a web-like covering that houses a nutmeg. Both can be used in cookery and in perfumery. However, nutmeg has a more subtle, sweet spiciness than cloves and cinnamon, for instance, and so tend to be used in masculine fragrances and light woodies. Mace is lighter still, with an almost milky spice note to its delicacy.

Found in:

Apparition - Ungaro

Kouros - Yves Saint Laurent

Very Irresistible - Givenchy

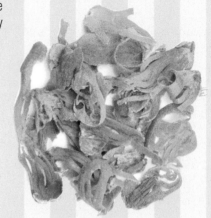

MAGNOLIA

Of all the plants this is one of the most ancient, as dinosaurs would have seen magnolia bloom in spring. Back then, though, they would have been pollinated by beetles rather than bees! You may also see Champaca listed, which is a yellow variety of magnolia.

The petals themselves have very little scent, so an absolute is made by solvent extraction. It is a highly valuable oil in skincare, but psychologically the extract is said to allow you to look and see your own inner beauty and then emanate it, so others fall in love with your spirit too—surely the real essence of perfume!

Found in:

Magnolia - Yves Rocher

Flora Glamorous Magnolia - Gucci

Heaven - Chopard

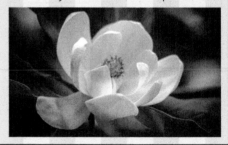

MANDARIN

Mandarin is the most hesperedic of notes. It is succulent, juicy, and sensuous; its fruit is a deliciously sweetish orange. It is possibly the sweetest and most uplifting of notes. The essential oil is obtained by expression of the rind of the fruit.

In Chinese medicine, you see it as having the yang energy of the sun—bright, positive and regenerative.

Found in:

Royal Peony Rose and Mandarin Musk - Lucy B

Mandarin Mist - Stila

212 Sexy Men - Carolina Herrera

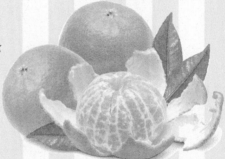

MARIGOLD

Predominately, the fragrance of marigold comes from the French marigold Tagetes. It has a rich, earthy, almost bitter scent to it. The name marigold comes from "Mary's Gold," which is the old name for the other marigold plant that is used in medicine, calendula. It is a pungent, strong, spicy floral note used in oriental fragrances.

Found in:

Eternity Love - Calvin Klein

Gatsby - Playboy

Halston Woman - Halston

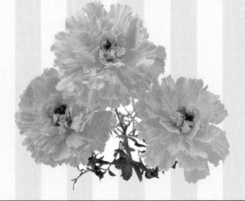

MIGNONETTE

As a Mediterranean herbaceous plant, mignonette is also known as Weld or Dyer's Rocket. Its root is used in natural dyes and can be traced back to the first millennium BC, which means it predates woad or madder.

Mignonette's violet-like, fruity, floral fragrance note was a particular favorite in Victorian society, not only in their perfumery but in potpourri as well to mask the less attractive environmental aromas.

Found in:

Montana Mood Sexy - Montana

Chanel No. 5 - Chanel

Aramis - Aramis

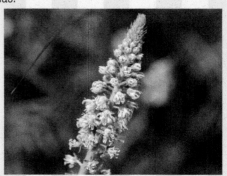

MIMOSA

One of perfumery's favorites, the diaphanous haziness of mimosa has the floral fragrance of genuine childlike innocence. It is sweet, soft and powdery, and floats gently to the top of oriental, chypre, and floral fragrance blends.

Many people associate it with yellow pom-pom flowers, which are in fact acacia, the cassie oil. Mimosa is a soft, dusky pink color, which resounds throughout the vibration of the oil.

Found in:

Mimosa - L'Erbolario

London - Burberry

Luna Rossa - Prada

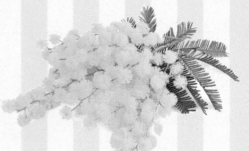

MYRRH

Always thought of in partnership with frankincense, the name myrrh means "bitter." It has a woody, earthy and pungent aroma to it. The resin which is generally used as incense can be made into two different perfumery components, an essential oil that is produced by distillation, and the more regularly used solvent extraction.

The deliciously resinous note of myrrh adds a robust edge to oriental and woody perfumes in particular.

In biblical times, myrrh was a spice commonly used for burials. It reference in the scriptures in the book of Esther and the Song of Solomon reflect another popular custom of laying a bundle of Myrrh on one's chest while sleeping as a beauty treatment in preparation for a wedding.

Myrrh was a highly-prized spice used for perfumes and incense, extracted by piercing the tree's heartwood and allowing the gum to trickle out and harden into bitter, aromatic red droplets called "tears." The Hebrew word for Myrrh is *mowr*, which means "distilled" and comes from the root word *marar*, which means "bitterness."

Myrrh serves as a fixing oil and enhances other fragrances in a blend.

Found in:

Myrrhiad - Paul Guillaume

Infusion de Tubereuse - Prada

Le Beau Male - Jean Paul Gaultier

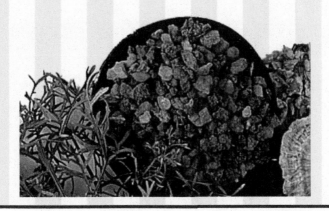

NARCISSUS

This beautiful, small daffodil has a sweet, hypnotic and heady floral note with a slightly green nuance to its fragrance. It has been a vital part of perfumery throughout history. The Romans used it to make a narcotic perfume called Narcissinum while the Arabs used it extensively and believed it could cure baldness.

The name narcissus stems from the Latin narc, which means "to become numb"—a poignant reminder of its narcotic reputation.

Narcissus is the world's most expensive absolute, requiring 500 kilograms of petals to make just one kilogram of concrete, which then translates to 300 grams of absolute. Today, production of the narcissus oil is restricted mainly to Grasse and some parts of the Netherlands.

Found in:

Romance Perfume - Ralph Lauren

Bouquet - Vera Wang

Polo - Ralph Lauren

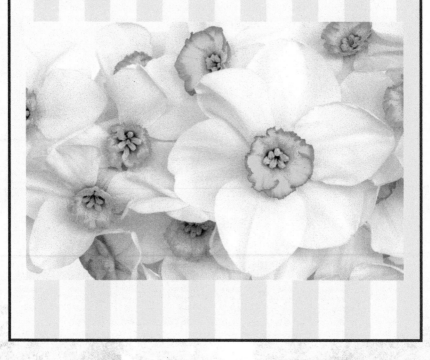

NEROLI

Neroli is made from the flowers of the bitter orange tree. Long having been the symbol of wedding day bliss, orange blossoms remind us of love and romance.

The bitter orange blooms offer up several products: bitter oranges themselves; petitgrain oil made from the leaves of the tree; neroli, which is obtained by distilling the flowers; and orange blossom, which is an absolute gained through solvent extraction.

Although taken from the same plant, the processes bring out very different characteristics of scent. Neroli is fresh and green, while the orange blossom is sweeter, headier, more like fresh flowers, and is commonly used in chypres and heavy orientals.

Found in:

Neroli - L'Occitane en Provence

Givenchy Harvest 2010 Organza Neroli for Women - Givenchy

Marbert Man Pure - Marbert

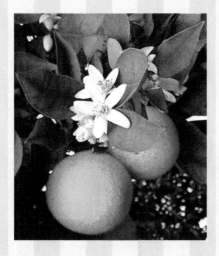

OAKMOSS

This inky, bitter-smelling moss is found growing beneath oak trees. The woody lichen has a woody, sharp and sensual tang to it. Oakmoss is invaluable to chypres and fougères. There is a different strain of the plant with a more turpentine hue that is also found under pines, and is revered in perfumery.

In 2001, the face of perfumery changed when restrictions were placed on the usage of oakmoss because of its sensitization potentials to the skin. Now, a total of no more than 0.1% of oakmoss and other tree mosses can be used in blends.

This ruling changed the recipes of many a wondrous fragrance, and the woody, exotic, deep forest edge was stolen away. Guerlain, feeling they could not continue without the freedom of the note, isolated the offending sensitizing constituent and was able to create a replacement without it. Thanks to modern science, this patented ingredient is 100% pure. Other fragrance houses took a different path, replacing oakmoss with vetiver or patchouli in their blends.

There are two oakmoss products. The first is a dark green resin that is solvent extracted and has an earthy, mossy note to it, almost like a leathery facet. The second is a vacuum distilled oakmoss, which is pale yellow and has a drier, earthier and more bark-like scent to it.

Found in:

Audace - Faberge

Constellation - Paloma Picasso

Aperçu - Houbigant

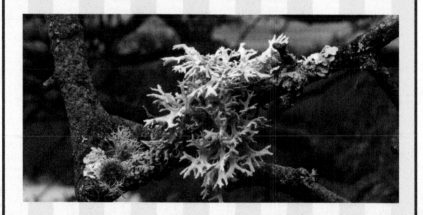

OPOPONAX

The resin tapped from the cousin of myrrh, opoponax also comes from the Commiphora family.

Where myrrh is bitter, opoponax is sweet, earthy and balsamic, and is utterly delicious. In the main, it is steam distilled but in fact can be extracted by any number of processes. It gives a sweet lift to chypre blends.

Found in:

Coco - Chanel

Opium - Yves Saint Laurent

Biagiotti Due Uomo - Laura Biagiotti

No. 8 Opopanax - Prada

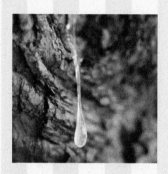

ORANGE BLOSSOM

The delicate flowers from the orange blossom produce this absolute. During the spring when the orange blossoms bloom, millions of delicate, waxy white flowers perfume the air as one of the most fragrant and indispensable materials in the perfume industry. Even though it comes from the same flower as neroli oil, it possesses different olfactory characteristics. The custom of a bride using fresh orange blossoms to decorate their hair on her wedding day became so widespread that the expression "to gather orange blossoms" took on the connotation to mean "to seek a wife."

Found in:

Lace Orange Flower for Women - Victoria's Secret

La Cologne Fleur du Male - Jean Paul Gaultier

APOM Pour Homme Maison for Men - Francis Kurkdjian

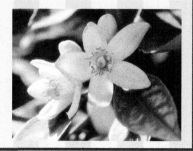

ORRIS

Orris is made from the roots of the iris plant. Orris has a distinctly different fragrance from the flower, and when separated takes on a deep, sweet and flowery aroma akin to violets.

In medieval times, it played a vital part in herbal medicine but now is only used in perfumery and as a fixative for incenses and potpourri.

Before use, the root is dried for five years and is then ground. The powder is dissolved in water and then is distilled. There is also an absolute occasionally used but is extremely pricey to produce needing one ton of powder to create two kilograms of the orris root butter.

Found in:

Fantasy - Britney Spears

Chanel No. 5 - Chanel

Noir Avon - Christian Lacroix

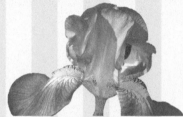

OSMANTHUS

This beautiful honey yellow to orange flowering bush is highly prized in the East but lesser known in the West. It is cultivated in China and then is exported to Grasse for producers to solvent extract using hexane into an absolute (a most expensive absolute, at that) with an exotic floral and oriental note.

It has a ripe fruitiness to it, the main scent being apricot, but there are undertones of ripe peaches and figs and a creamy, leathery nuance too.

It is well recognized for bringing about happiness and smiles, and because of this, the flowers are often added to tea in China. The description makes it feel like a heart note, but osmanthus is a clearly chiming top note in blends.

Found in:

Nuance - Roberto Capucci

Flowerbomb Extreme Sparkle 2008 - Viktor & Rolf

Les Nombres d'Or Oud - Mona di Orio

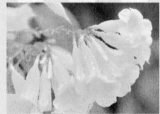

PALMAROSA

This rosy scented oil actually comes from a grass that is a member of the lemongrass family. The oil is extremely high in geraniol, which is what gives it its flowery fragrance, and is often used to "cut" rose oils, especially in Turkey.

It is native to India, and while mainly grown for distillation into an essential oil, it is also used by grain and bean crop farmers as an insect repellent.

The fragrance is bright and sunshiny, with a geranium scent on a summer's morning.

Palmarosa is popular for adding a less costly yet tenacious rose-geranium like scent to your perfume blends. As a middle to top note, it is often used as an ingredient in soaps, cosmetics, and in the flavoring of tobacco.

Found in:

The Party in Paris - The Party

Geranium Bourbon - Miller Harris

Notas para dos Energy - Bottega Verde

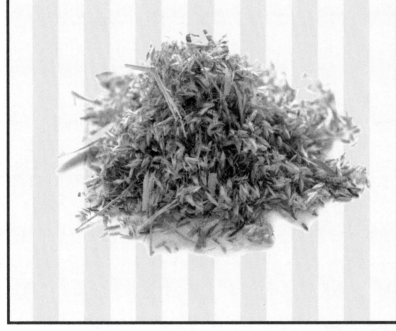

PATCHOULI

A most misunderstood oil, patchouli is often associated with the synthetic, overly sweet edition worn by hippies and bikers in the 1960s and 70s. In its natural form, it has a stirring woody earthiness to it, and yes, it is sweet but has a delicious balsamic and sensuous touch to it.

Originally brought to the West by Napoleon, he carried two beautifully ornate scarves from Egypt, which had been imbued with patchouli to repel insects. For many years, work took place replicating the intricate patterns of the stoles, but the redolent fragrance was kept a closely guarded secret and was imported to finish the valuable package deal. It was not until 1837 when Francisco Manuel described patchouli as Menta cablin that the secret was discovered.

Many people are surprised to find it comes from the green leaves of a variety of mint. The oil is made with great care, collected from only the top three or four pairs of leaves of the plant, where the oil concentration is highest.

The leaves are carefully laid upon boards and repeatedly turned to dry and then are placed in baskets to ferment. The producer's nose determines the exact point where fermentation is correct, and then the dried leaves are either steam distilled or CO2 extracted.

Both are used in perfumery, but the CO2 version is more balsamic with a more minty undertone clearly perceived.

Found in:

Surreal Garden - Avon

Kate - Kate

H&M - Comme des Garcons

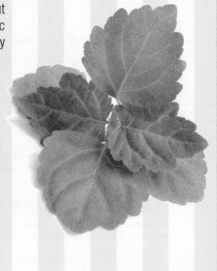

PENNYROYAL

Used much by the ancient Greeks and Romans, Pennyroyal has somewhat gone out of fashion. It is a member of the mint family but differs from most as the leaves grow in curly whorls around the stem. It has a fresh aromatic note to it but is closer to that of spearmint than peppermint.

Found in:

Pheromone - Marilyn Miglin

Hello Kitty - Hello Kitty

Halston Men - Halston

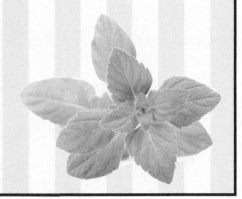

PEPPERMINT

The best known of the mint family, this is a fresh, clear aromatic note that adds a bracing dimension to a perfume. The essential oil is extracted by steam distillation from the leaves of the plant.

The plant, dating back to around 1500 BC, is believed to be a hybrid of water mint and spearmint. It is seen in various recipes found in ancient Egypt, and was a well traded herb. In the book of Luke, we read how Jesus scorned the Pharisees for placing their love of trading mint in the courts of the temple above their love of the Lord.

Found in:

Mint - Toni Gard

Oriental Mint - Phaedon

Police - Original

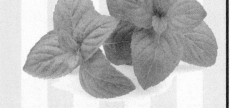

PETITGRAIN

Obtained from the bitter orange tree, petitgrain is steam distilled from the leaves and twigs. Although taken from the same plant as neroli and sweet orange, petitgrain has an aroma profile all of its own. It has a slightly rosy zing to it and, of course, a very woody note.

Petitgrain is often found in florals and colognes.

Found in:

Dior Addict - Dior

Chakra 3 Equipoise - Aveda

Mister Marvelous - Redo

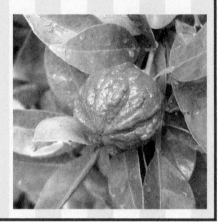

PINE NEEDLE

The fresh, woody and slightly astringent fragrance of pine are more often found in men's fragrances than women's. There are, of course, exceptions. The oil is derived by steam distillation from the needles as well as the wood of the pine tree, of which there are 115 different species.

The majority of oil is obtained from the United States and Hungary where pine trees grow prolifically. It is a well cultivated crop as it is a favorite in construction, not least because of its immunity to decay and insects after logging.

The woody aromatic note of pine needles is often found in fougères.

Found in:

Private Collection - Estée Lauder

Eau Jeune Double Je - Eau Jeune

Pi Leather Jacket - Givenchy

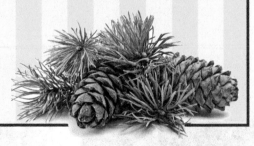

ROSE

The fundamental component of any floral scent brings a rose to mind. It comes in two forms: rose otto, which is achieved by distillation, and rose absolute. Otto is lighter and more ethereal than the deep, sultry absolute. The two variations are as different to one another in vibration as night and day.

The sweetly spicy oil is extremely costly to produce despite its full-bodied scent in the natural bloom. A significant number of petals are needed to produce even the smallest amount of oil. Although a very feminine note, rose will often be found adding sweetness and lightness to men's blends too.

Found in:

Joy - Jean Patou

Bvlgari Pour Femme - Bvlgari

Rose Oud - Kilian

ROSE DE MAI

Rose de Mai comes from the breed Rosa x centifolia (quite literally "the rose of a hundred petals"), also called cabbage rose. The hybrid was developed around the eighteenth century by Dutch breeders who crossed Rosas gallica, damascena, moschata, and canina. The result is a stunningly lovely bloom with an unyielding fragrance of sweetness and honey. It is clear and almost hypnotic.

The best place to see Rose de Mai in all its glory is in Grasse, France where they create the most spectacular absolute for use in floral and oriental perfumes.

Found in:

Satin Rose de Mai - Victoria's Secret

Fleurs de Jontue - Revlon

French Rose - Fragonard

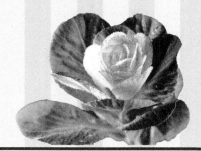

ROSEMARY

An aromatic note taken from the well recognized herb from our kitchens. It has a rustic romance to it. Historically, it is an important part of perfumery as it was one of the main components of Hungary Water, the first alcohol-based perfume in Europe made by Elisabeth of Poland during the fourteenth century.

It comes from the Lamiaceae family, the mint family, and indeed it has a sharp, camphorous, astringent flavor to it.

One will find rosemary verbenone a softer, gentler version to the more common and pungent cineole variety. Its refreshing and herbaceous nature brings warmth with mildiy sweet qualities to a fragrance.

Found in:

Egoiste - Chanel

Pi - Givenchy

Paco Rabanne - Paco Rabanne

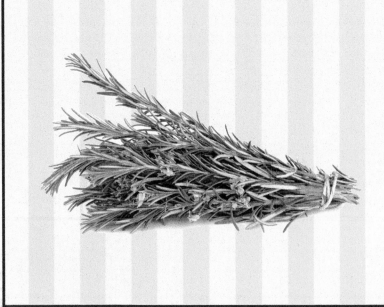

SANDALWOOD

Sandalwood has been treasured for over 4,000 years in India and is closely linked with their beliefs about fertility. The sapwood of the tree is white, but the heartwood is much revered for its rich, bright yellow-red color and rich scent of oil. Often wood that is carved continues to emanate the oil's fragrance for many years to come.

The very best oil is taken from the sandalwood mysore, which is grown in India but sadly has been harvested almost to the point of extinction. Since sandalwood is a slow-growing crop, mysore is now under protection, and most sandalwood essential oil comes from the most sustainable resources of Australia and New Caledonia.

The profile of this substitute oil does not have the creaminess of its rich, sweet, balsamic note of mysore. Still incredibly sensuous, though, these more available oils have a harsher edge to them—and somehow, they have a greener top to them.

Sandalwood is a base note used in many blends but is of particular importance in oriental, chypre and woody blends.

Found in:

Samsara - Guerlain

Hypnotic Poison - Dior

Oliban - Phaedon

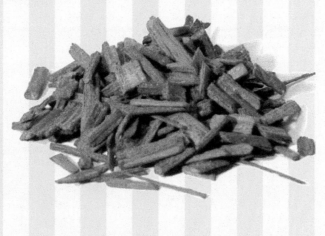

SIBERIAN FIR

Essential oils are extracted by distillation from not only Siberian but also Balsamic and White firs. Collected from the needles, each has their own aroma profile. White fir is the sweetest of the three. Balsamic is as you would expect, more balsamic, and Siberian fir has the same edge but is more woody and sharper than the others. They each are like fresh air in your lungs and are incredibly delightful. Siberian fir is the most commonly used of the three in perfumery. It belongs to the woody olfactory group.

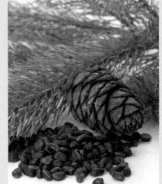

Found in:

Rocabar - Hermes

Green Jeans - Versace

Les Parfums Mythiques - Givenchy

STAR ANISE

Not to be confused with anise (or aniseed), star anise has a harder, more bitter-scented profile than its similarly named compatriot. It is steam distilled from the fresh or partly dried star-shaped pods and seeds of the spice we recognize from Asian cooking. Its silky, licorice-like, deep, rich scent gives an exotic lilt to oriental blends and balances out the sweetness of floral fragrances. Star anise is a gorgeously sultry oriental note.

Found in:

Classique - Jean Paul Gaultier

Loverdose - Diesel

Rosa Centifolia de Chateauneuf de Grasse - Givenchy

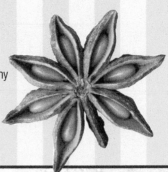

SWEET ORANGE

The orange we know today is a hybrid between a pomelo and a mandarin, which was first cultivated in southern China during the eleventh century. By the fifteenth century, Italian traders had spread seeds around the globe, and today the orange is the world's most common tree fruit.

Sweet orange's scent inevitably requires no description. Its hesperedic sweet note has a deliciously astringent tartness to it. The citrus note of orange can be found as a bright top note in all types of perfumes.

Found in:

Hidden Fantasy - Brittany Spears

Woman Number 1 - Betty Barclay

Happy Smile - Clinique

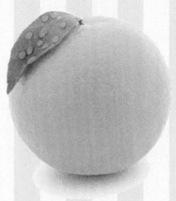

TANGERINE

The tangerine is a subspecies of the mandarin family. It takes its name from the port of Tangiers in Morocco from whence it was first exported in 1841.

Smaller than a standard orange, it is heavy with juice, but the essential oil itself is expressed from the rind of the fruit.

It has a sweeter, more honeyed note than orange, and its citrus note doesn't seem to have quite the zingy sharpness either. It is a delicately happy ingredient found particularly in citrus fragrances, of course, and in oriental blends too.

Found in:

Fan di Fendi - Fendi

Fraiche Badione Maitre - Parfumeur et Gantiers

Jump Hot Summer - Joop!

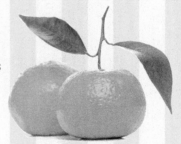

TEA

The refreshing taste of tea is recognized and loved around the world. The leaves of the *Camellia sinensis*, however, do not give up their scents easily. They are extracted by CO2 to make absolutes. Just as there are many types of tea, so there are many absolutes.

Green tea is a sticky semi-solid concoction that has a fresh apricot note with a woody undertone. It adds a full-bodied heart note to florals and citrus accords in particular.

Black tea absolute has the look of thick molten molasses and has the bitter smokiness we associate with tea.

The absolute of maté is intense and has a similar reminiscence to hay that we expect from coumarins. Often this note lends depth to fougères creations. Rooibosch is rarely produced, and blends requiring this note are often created using a tincture.

Found in:

Aroma Tonique - Lancôme

Wish of Peace - Avon

Thé Vert - Roger and Gallet

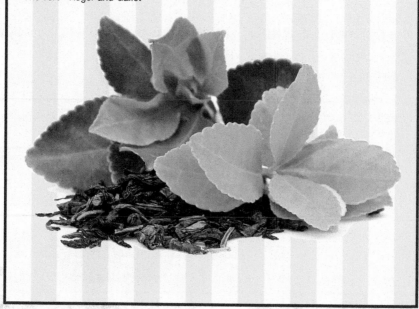

TONKA BEAN

This oriental note is one of the most valuable in perfumery. This is the source of a hay-like scented component called coumarin. It is extracted from the wrinkled black seeds of the Diptery odorata, which were introduced to France in 1793 from South America. To this day, Brazil and Venezuela continue to be the largest producers of the extract.

The tropical tree has beautiful purple flowers with scents of vanilla, saffron and cinnamon that float for miles on the breeze. Inside of each flower is a bean.

These beans are dried and then soaked for twelve hours in rum until white crystals of coumarin collect on the outside of the bean. The extract is not runny, but is quite solid, but can be made more malleable with the application of heat. In fact, technically it is not an essential oil nor an absolute and has no classification of its own.

However, coumarin has been found to cause dreadful liver damage, so the ingredient (that often was used as a substitute for vanilla) is banned in many parts of the world. Coumarin with its scent of newly mown hay crossed with almonds is now made synthetically.

Found in:

Coco - Chanel

Diversity - Mexx

Shalimar - Guerlain

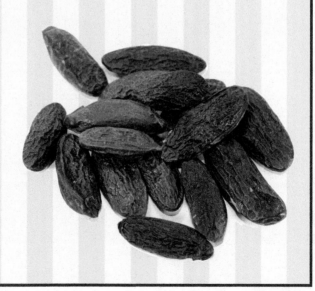

TUBEROSE

The strangest of all the floral notes, tuberose has a mentholated freshness to it at the beginning when the flowers bloom, but as it ripens it becomes almost redolent of rotting meat. With that said, tuberose is either loved or abhorred. Its loose profile is heady, carnal and slattern; indeed Victorian girls were forbidden from smelling the blooms for fear of what might happen.

The strong fragrance tempted perfumers to capture the essence through the costly method of effleurage as early as the seventeenth century, but the fact it requires 1,200 kilograms of unopened buds to create just 200 milliliters of absolute makes it a difficult ingredient to use in perfumery.

For this reason, most tuberose used in blends is now synthetically produced. This is also an opportunity to capture the facets of the plant producers want to emulate. Some bring forward the creaminess and highlight the menthol tones, perhaps, or for more brazen blends maybe the depth of the ripened decay seems more appropriate.

Found in:

Amarige - Givenchy

Fracas - Robert Piguet

Passage No. 9 - Dior

TURMERIC

The rich, warm earthy spice of turmeric is taken from the root of the plant. Instantly recognizable by the aroma of curry, turmeric tends to be used mostly in oriental blends but more often in masculine fragrances.

The plant, also known as Indian saffron, has huge green leaves and exotic-looking red blooms. It loves the dry and arid ground, and somehow this warm, dusty, parched feel comes through in its profile. This has an invigorating accord, sizzling in its sensuality.

Found in:

Eau de Narcisse - Hermes

Tommy Hilfiger - Tommy Hilfiger

8 88 - Comme Des Garcons

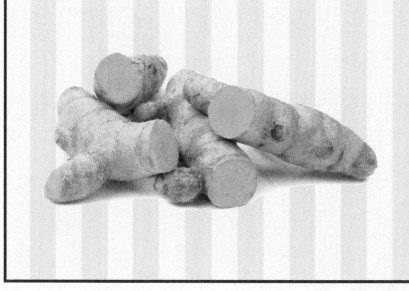

VANILLA

This popular oriental fragrance note is synonymous with cookies and ice cream. It is extracted from a type of orchid with its natural extract being expensive to produce. In its pure form, it is magically deep, rich and velvety, almost treacle-like, warming and cozy. It was rediscovered in the West when it was brought back from the Americas in the seventeenth century, but the Native Indian had long since revered the spice. The Aztecs blended it into chocolate for their most exotic of royal drinks, called Tlilxochitl.

Vanilla is not available as an essential oil, but rather an absolute. As extraction is so expensive, there are very few real extracts available. For this reason, the synthetic variant vanillin is often used as a replacement in perfume.

One will find rosemary verbenone a softer, gentler version to the more common and pungent cineole variety. Its refreshing and herbaceous nature brings warmth with mildiy sweet qualities to a fragrance.

Found in:

Shalimar - Guerlain

Hypnose - Lancôme

Vanilla Musk - Coty

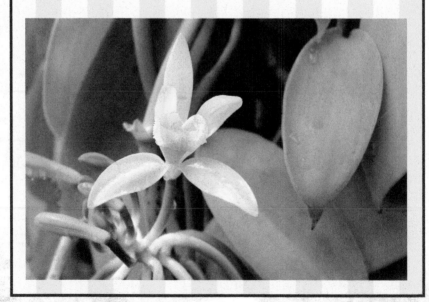

VANILLIN

The principle constituent that gives its scent to vanilla is vanillin, which is now synthesized for use in perfumery. The process for replication has gone through many alterations through time. In 1858, Nicolas Theodor Gobley obtained a vanillin extract by drying a vanilla bean and then soaking the solids in hot water.

Later in 1874, German scientists were able to isolate its chemical structure and managed to synthesize it using pine bark. By the end of nineteenth century, it had become possible to replicate it from clove oil. By the 1930s, vanillin had become a commercially and viable component. Vanillin found its place in perfumery, used predominately in chypres and orientals but not exclusively.

Scentwise, vanillin does not have the balsamic earthiness of vanilla. Instead, its scent is more the aroma of vanilla essence.

Found in:

Shalimar - Guerlain

Jicky - Guerlain

Prima Dulcis - Arquiste

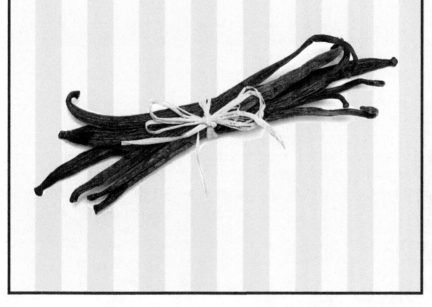

VERBENA

Lemon verbena is both a citrus and an aromatic note. It is extracted by distillation from the rough green leaves of the plant, which had originally been discovered in Buenos Ares in 1767. At a time when plant smuggling was rife, samples of the plant were impounded from a stash gathered by French botanist Joseph Dombey during an eight-year stay in Lima. The plants were left to rot in greenhouses in Cadiz, and many of the samples in his collection were lost. Lemon verbena survived, however, and seeds were then brought to France and England. It has become a flavoring favorite in teas and with fish, but also for its wonderful scent in potpourri.

The essential oil is obtained by distillation from the young leaves. The note gives a lemony green top note to fragrances.

Found in:

Green Irish Tweed - Creed

Jasper Conran II Man - Jasper Conran

Pure - DKNY

VETIVER

This coarse, dried grass from India has long been loved for its cooling aroma. In India, blinds were made from vetiver to keep out the intense heat and would be splashed with water to release their subtle fragrance. In Java, mats are woven to welcome and cool visitors who find their way to one's doorstep.

It is a musty, wood note, somewhere between bitter chocolate and wood smoke. As it dries down, it takes on a leathery-amber note.

The essential oil, which is distilled from the dried blades of the grass, is a well-used component in perfumery. Its cooling qualities contribute to 36% of Western scents for women and 20% of men's fragrances.

Found in:

Encre Noir - Lalique

Velvet Vetivert - Dolce & Gabanna

Chypre - Coty

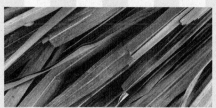

VIOLET

The violet plant lends us two products. The essence of the flower has an earthy, powdery and sweet aroma while the leaves have a greener, more metallic note. The floral fragrance that you would recognize as parma violets is due to a component called ionones. This is what is responsible for the woody sweetness.

In 1896, the discovery of this constituent made it possible to isolate the component and replicate it. Because of the costly nature of extracting violet essence, the synthetic version is almost always used.

It is often found as a floral note in richly sweet perfumes. The leaf, however, also has its place in perfumery as a woody note and is extracted as an absolute.

Found in:

Ultraviolet - Paco Rabanne

Violet Precieusse - Caron

Fahrenheit - Dior

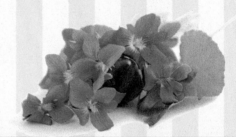

YLANG YLANG

The Canaga odorata is from Madagascar originally, but it is now naturalized in Malaysia and Burma. Ylang ylang oil is steam distilled from the petals of its yellow blooms, which prompted its name meaning "Flower of flowers."

There are two types of this plant: a tree and a vine. The vines especially have wondrous flowers that are almost sickly sweet, spicy and exotic. These become even more fragrant and have an almost narcotic air to them once evening comes.

Found in:

Amarige - Givenchy

My Ylang - Caron

Chanel No. 5 - Chanel

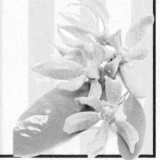

AMBERGRIS

Ambergris was, for centuries, believed to be some kind of mythical wonder as the gray, exotically fragranced ingredient would wash up unexplainably on shores. Its wonderful perfume and its fixative qualities for other scents made it highly prized and sought after by merchants across the globe.

We now know it comes from the sperm whale who regurgitates it after eating cuttlefish or squid whose bones irritate the whale's stomach lining; ambergris is the counter attack to this. The trade of ambergris now falls under the Protected Species Act and is largely banned; thus, ambergris has to be replaced by a synthetic replica.

When first created, natural ambergris (literally translated as gray amber) has a strong fecal stench but over time softens to a sweet, earthy smell. The ancient Egyptians burned it as incense and in medieval times people carried around a ball of it to chase away the reek of the Black Plague which they feared was the carrier of the disease.

Found in:

L'eau Ambrée - Prada

Dioressence - Dior

Eau de Merveilles - Hermes

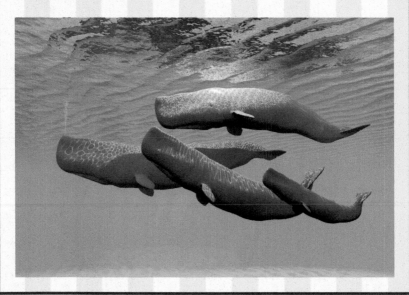

CASTOREUM

This is now entirely made synthetically, a copy of the secretion from the castor sacs of beavers. The rich, dark leathery scent is lusty, brazen and passionate. For many generations, the beaver has been hunted, not only for castoreum but also for their waterproof fur and their flavorsome meat. As a consequence, by the sixteenth century, beavers could no longer be found in Scotland. Despite this, the bright, burning fragrance was still used in perfumery until the early twentieth century.

Found in:

Amouge - Epic Man

Antaeus - Chanel

Paloma Picasso - Paloma Picasso

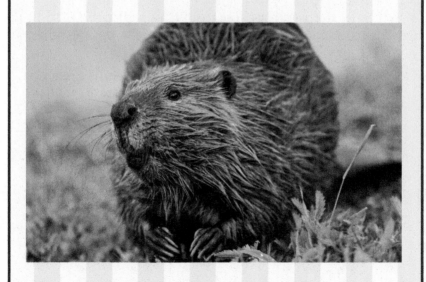

CIVET

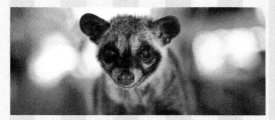

The musk-like pheromone is secreted by a catlike creature by the same name to mark his territory. So prized in history, it was cited as a gift given to impress the Queen of Sheba and held the trading value of gold, frankincense, and ivory.

The secretion is rich with animalistic passion and has long been one of the most sought-after accords in a fragrance blend. In the 1940s it was discovered how to synthesize the note, and for the most part, this engineered version is what is used in blends.

However, this is not always used. In Ethiopia, there are farmers who rely on the trade of civet oil for their livelihood. Reserved for trade only allowed to Muslims, silviculture is alive and well. Legend has it the much-loved leader Nessiru Allah declared that followers of the religion should always farm the African civet after his eye affliction was miraculously healed using an application of it.

It is erroneously presumed the animals are killed for the trade, but in fact, the creatures are kept caged for their next secretion. The amounts produced by the beasts are minuscule but regular so their lives sadly can be long and incredibly stressful.

Today, for the most part, civetone is used and is synthesized from palm oil. It would seem this is a good copy as reports state camera traps are baited with Calvin Klein's Obsession for Men to get the very best footage of jaguars.

Found in:

Joy - Jean Patou

Shalimar - Guerlain

Jicky - Guerlain

This does not imply real civet is still used in these blends.

HYRAX

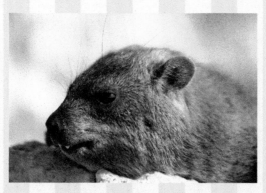

It is refreshing among this list of upsetting practices to talk about the small rodent, the hyrax. This small shrew-like rodent lives in Africa, and strangely is the elephant's closest living relative. Only 20-30 centimeters long, it resembles a guinea pig but does maintain some of the elephant's features, such as the fact that the male's scrotum is hidden inside of the mammal by the kidney. Their tusks, like an elephant, are developed from the incisor teeth.

Archaeological evidence shows hyrax scurried around the earth as early as 40 million years ago. Perhaps they did not scurry, though, as it is suspected in those days the hyrax was as large as a horse—closer than to an elephant, perhaps!

In perfumery, hyrax, sometimes known as hyraceum, is used. The hyrax marks its territory over and over again with a gel-like substance. Because the animal has a small territory, it is easy to find large amounts of the substance in a small vicinity. The substance used in perfumery is the fossilized and petrified gel.

Now hardened by millions of years, the stone like substance is ground and then added to denatured alcohol to release its musky, almost tobacco-like fragrance.

Found in:

Ayala Moriel - Bouquet of Love

Espirit du Rio - Penhaligans

Fils de Dieu du riz et des Argumes - Etat Libre d'Orange

MUSK

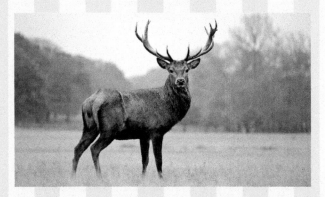

The scent source of all desire comes from the pheromones secreted by the male musk deer. The small creature has two glands under his belly called pods which he uses to secrete the musk to attract his mate.

Sadly, the deer is hunted to take the pods and collect the musk; it is predicted that as many as 60,000 musk deer are killed to smuggle out 450 grams of musk. Most of the musk goes to followers of traditional medicine for its myriad of uses, but mainly for its aphrodisiac effects.

As recently as the 1980s, fragrance houses in Western Europe and Japan were still using musk extensively. In 1999, however, the European Union banned the import of musk, forcing the industry to use synthetic versions.

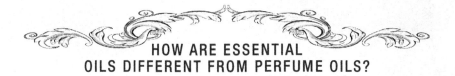

HOW ARE ESSENTIAL
OILS DIFFERENT FROM PERFUME OILS?

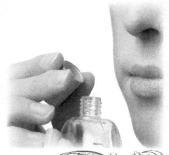

*E*ssential oils are very concentrated extracts from stems, wood, flowers, buds, resins, leaves, and bark. These are great for making perfumes, but can be too intense to be directly applied to the skin. In contrast, perfume oils are fragrances that have been suspended in an oil base. They may be natural or synthetically produced. Perfume oils are safe to apply to the skin.

PERFUMER'S ALCOHOL VERSUS FORMULATOR'S ALCOHOL

Most of us are familiar with alcohol in some form. But did you know that there are different types of alcohol used in perfumery? The most common ones used in perfume making is formulator's alcohol and perfumer's alcohol. Let's take a look at the characteristics and uses of these two forms of alcohol.

FORMULATOR'S ALCOHOL

Formulator's alcohol is usually found in household products such as air fresheners and linen sprays; this product is mild and doesn't cause any adverse allergic reactions. This substance may also be found in liquor and is ingestible. Also, some people use it for faster fermentation of yeast, which can then be used to prepare bread.

Formulator's alcohol naturally exists by itself. It has an average purity rate of 75%, while its counterparts contain only 30-40% of the original substance. It is available at professional liquor vendors. Formulator's alcohol is odorless. However, it cannot be mixed with other substances to form a positive reaction. This is because of its mild fundamental nature. Formulator's alcohol is one of the most versatile types of alcohol and has many beneficial uses.

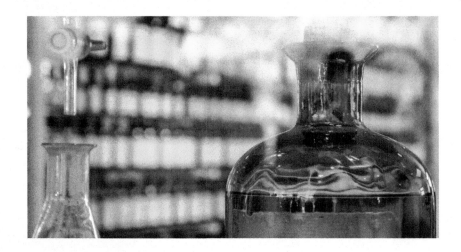

Formulator's alcohol has been found to help fragrances last much longer, as it contains synthesizers that improve aroma and slow down the rate of evaporation, especially when out in the open. This unique alcohol also provides a layer of protection when mixed with essential oils, thus ensuring it stays fresh throughout the day without mingling with perspiration.

Formulator's alcohol blends well with substances such as resinous, sticky oils, benzoin, orris, and vetiver. These are natural scents with an earthy appeal that deepen when the alcohol is added. Store formulator's alcohol in a dark place away from direct sunlight, preferably in a cool cabinet, to protect it from evaporation.

PERFUMER'S ALCOHOL
Perfumer's alcohol is specially formulated to maximize and hold onto the scent of fragrances. The substance may also be used in the production of diffuser oils, where it usually makes the blended solution remain spotlessly clean and free from cloudiness. Perfumer's alcohol consists of three sub-ingredients. These compounds include denatured ethanol, which acts as the primary carrier ingredient in fragrance oils; it easily evaporates when warmed by one's skin temperature and uniformly distributes fragrances around the surface. Isopropyl myristat helps in the absorption of essential

oils and fragrances into the alcoholic solution. Monopropylene glycol is a co-solvent product that allows fragrance oil constituents to be solubilized into the alcohol carrier. The process helps in controlling the rate of evaporation so that the alcohol doesn't fade away too quickly.

Perfumer's alcohol contains an extra ingredient, which allows other substances to mix nicely and permanently. It can easily support a ratio of 66% alcohol and 33% pure perfume oil. Perfumer's alcohol is a great choice since it settles down easily and sustains the skin's lustrous nature.

USES OF PERFUMER'S ALCOHOL AND FORMULATOR'S ALCOHOL

Perfumer's alcohol can be used in making homemade fragrances in a more professional way. One reason is that it makes a nice solvent even when mixed with resinous oils. You can also blend it with absolutes, isolated aromatic chemicals, and organic scents. When added to absolutes, it makes the substance smell stronger and more appealing than just essential oils; it can thus be used in custom perfumery processes. Moreover, some scented plants are very delicate and can hardly be steam distilled or pressed to remove the essential oils found inside; the jasmine flower is one such example. However, perfumer's alcohol is easier to process even from home.

On the other hand, formulator's alcohol helps in the synthesis of aroma chemicals, which are either synthetically produced or refined in the lab. An example is a compound known as vanillin, which gives vanilla ice cream its classic characteristic scent and flavor. Artificial vanilla used for making flavored liquor is usually synthetic and produced by mixing it with formulator's alcohol. This helps in smoothing up the vanilla extracts and releasing a sweet and safe aroma.

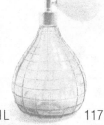

ESSENTIAL OILS AND ABSOLUTES

Chapter 6

UNDERSTANDING NOTES

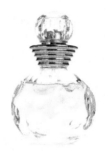

The next step will be for him (the beginner) to establish a classification of odorous materials according to their volatility. While such a classification could be established scientifically, the apprentice perfumer will soon attain unexpected proficiency by forgetting technical information he/she may have, and by establishing "his/her" classification for him/herself, as I had to 40 years ago.

– JEAN CARLES,
LEGENDARY TWENTIETH CENTURY PERFUMER

Imagine your aromatic blend is a musical composition, and you are writing a masterpiece. This is how a famous perfumer, Septimus Piesse, described it. Fragrant oils and their odors have been compared to sounds or musical notes. Just like a musical scale, going from the first or lowest note to last or highest note, scents range from the heavy smells up to the sharpest smell.

Perfume is seldom made with just one fragrance. They are usually a blend of up to three or more fragrances, consisting of base notes, middle notes, and top notes.

Edward Sagarin, the author of *The Science and Art of Perfumery* (New York, NY: McGraw-Hill, 1945), wrote, "Another contribution to the field of odor classification was made by the famous perfumer and perfume historian, Septimus Piesse. This unique figure in the history of science created what he called the 'odophone.' The odors were like sounds, he pointed out, and a scale could be created going from the first or lowest note, the heavy smell to the last or highest note, the sharp smell. In between, there was an ascending ladder. Each odor note corresponded to a key on his odophone, and in the creation of a happy mixture of many different odors, which we call a 'bouquet' and which every finished perfume must be, the creator seeks not only to hit the right notes but to strike those notes which go with one another. His perfume must not be out of tune."

Your perfume will contain one or more from each of the above categories: a base note, middle note, and top note. Some perfumers recommend using a four note, called a bridge note.

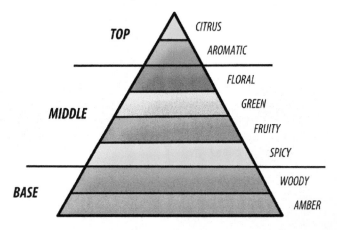

TOP NOTES (HEAD) are oils that have a light, fresh aroma. These are the first scents you smell after applying a blend to the skin. Although they quickly evaporate, the top note is what gives us our first impression of a blend. Common top notes include eucalyptus, lemon, bergamot, orange, lime and other citrus oils. In fact, bergamot is one of the most widely used essential oils in the perfumery and toiletry industry, together with neroli and lavender, as the main ingredients for the classical eau-de-cologne fragrance.

Most top notes are made up chemically of aldehydes and esters, which are generally found in oils from fruits, flowers, and leaves.

MIDDLE NOTES (HEART) also referred to as heart notes are usually the inspiration for an aromatic blend or perfume and include floral scents such as geranium, Roman chamomile, lavender, or neroli. It is generally considered the heart of the blend as it often serves to cover up any unpleasant scents that may come from the base notes. Essential oils classified as middle notes are sometimes referred to as enhancers, equalizers, or balancers. Chemically, these are monoterpene alcohols found mostly in herbs and leaves. Examples of essential oil middle notes include lavender, Roman chamomile, cypress, geranium, juniper berry, rosemary, and peppermint. Middle notes are what we smell when the scent from the top notes fades. This scent often evaporates after 15 seconds. The middle note can play on the emotions, and are often found in flowers, leaves, and needles. They act to bring together the top and base notes as the "synergy" in a blend.

BOTTOM NOTES (BASE) are usually the backbone and foundation of the blend and are what the users will remember most about the particular fragrance. The scent of base notes will last the longest in the air and are what you smell after about 30 seconds of applying it to your skin. The base note is added to the mixture first. Examples of essential oil base notes include vanilla, sandalwood, patchouli, frankincense, lichens, cinnamon, and other earthy and woodsy scents. Typically, a perfume has at least one base note oil in it, as it will stay the longest on the skin. Aromatic blends can have one or more base oils to add character.

Chemically speaking, base notes are made up of sesquiterpenes or diterpenes and are mainly found in roots, gums, and resins. Perfumes may contain one or more base notes. However, for any blend to be balanced, they must have a combination of all three notes.

When blending by note, it is crucial to add the extracts in order starting with the base note, followed by the middle note and finally the top note. This ensures your blend will create a wonderful aroma known as a "bouquet" by staying in tune with odor intensity as well as finding notes that strike a chord and harmonize well together aromatically.

The following chart, Classification of Essential Oils by Notes, lists the most popular essential oils by their common name and note classification: Top, Middle, or Base. Please note, some oils made fall into more than one category. For example, lemongrass is listed as a top note and middle note. This is possible because of the many components essential oils possess and the synergy effect a blend might draw out of that oil. For this reason, you may find perfumers disagree on which group they fall in. However, don't let this trouble you. Instead, let this work to your advantage when creating your blends. For instance, there may come a time when you have several middle note essential oils on hand to choose from, but no top notes for your particular recipe. In this case, you could use lemongrass as your top note and choose a different oil as your middle note. Follow this simply as a guide when orchestrating your blends and let your nose have the final say.

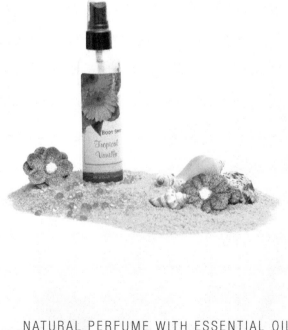

CLASSIFICATION OF ESSENTIAL OILS BY NOTES

TOP	MIDDLE	BASE
Ajowan	Allspice	Angelica Root
Aniseed	Ambrette Seed	Balsam
Anise Star	Balsam Fir	Benzoin
Basil	Bay	Spikenard
Bay Laurel	Black Pepper (to base)	Cedarwood
Bergamot	Blue Tansy	Cistus Labdanum
Birch	Cananga	Davana
Cajeput	Caraway Seed	Frankincense
Camphor	Cardamom (to top)	Ginger
Cedar Leaf	Carrot Seed	Helichrysum
Citronella	Cassia	Jasmine
Clary Sage (to middle)	Chamomile	Myrrh
Coriander	Cinnamon	Oakmoss
Eucalyptus	Clove Bud	Opoponax
Fennel (to middle)	Cumin	Patchouli
Fleabane (to middle)	Cypress (to base)	Rose
Galbanum	Dill	Rosewood
Garlic	Douglas Fir	Sandalwood
Grapefruit	Elemi	Tarragon
Lemon	Fir Needle	Turmeric
Lemon Myrtle	Geranium	Valerian
Lemongrass (to middle)	Gingergrass	Vanilla
Lime	Goldenrod	Vetiver
Mandarin	Ho Wood	Violet Leaf (to middle)
May Chang	Hyssop (to top)	Wormwood
Orange, Sweet	Inula	Ylang Ylang (to middle)
Orange, Bitter	Juniper Berry	
Oregano	Lavandin	

TOP	MIDDLE	BASE
Palo Santo	Lavender	
Peppermint (to middle)	Linaloe Berry	
Petitgrain	Marjoram	
Ravensara (to middle)	Melissa (to top)	
Sage (to middle)	Myrtle (to top)	
Scotch Pine	Neroli (to top)	
Spearmint	Niaouli	
Tangerine	Nutmeg	
Tea Tree	Palmarosa	
Tulsi	Parsley	
Verbena, Lemon	Pimento Leaf	
	Pine	
	Plai	
	Ravintsara	
	Rosalina	
	Rose Geranium	
	Rosemary	
	Spruce	
	Tagetes (to top)	
	Thyme (to top)	
	Wild Tansy	
	Winter Savory	
	Wintergreen	
	Xanthoxylum	
	Yarrow	

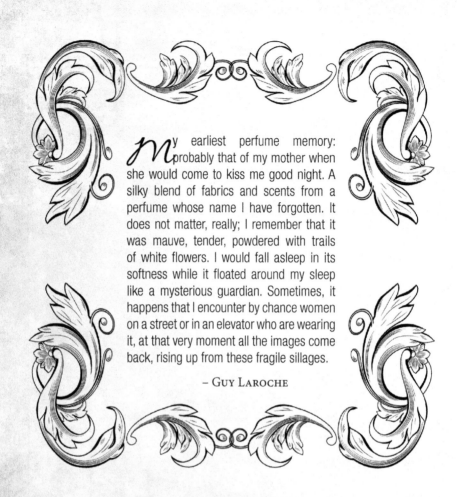

My earliest perfume memory: probably that of my mother when she would come to kiss me good night. A silky blend of fabrics and scents from a perfume whose name I have forgotten. It does not matter, really; I remember that it was mauve, tender, powdered with trails of white flowers. I would fall asleep in its softness while it floated around my sleep like a mysterious guardian. Sometimes, it happens that I encounter by chance women on a street or in an elevator who are wearing it, at that very moment all the images come back, rising up from these fragile sillages.

– GUY LAROCHE

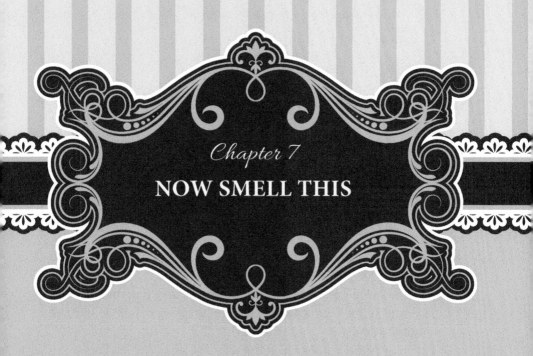

Chapter 7

NOW SMELL THIS

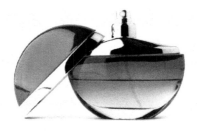

*Olfactory training is of prime importance,
and should never be neglected or interrupted.
Our own perfumers make it a strict rule to test,
daily, their knowledge of perfume materials,
and this is why a half hour is set apart for
this exercise.*

– JEAN CARLES,
LEGENDARY TWENTIETH CENTURY PERFUMER

In this chapter, you will be evaluating the composition of your individual essential oils to become familiar with their components. Practice by starting with one essential oil you have on hand to learn more about its volatility rate. This will allow you to see how it evaporates during the drydown, revealing its top note, middle note, and base note, and become more familiar with its character.

1. Take out all of your oils in a clean work area. Using your perfume strips or blotters, write the name of the essential oil on one end of the thin strip.
2. Note the time and date on the strip and write "#1" on it.
3. Dip the other end of the strip into your oil and fan the blotter about 3-5 inches below your nose and take a short, light whiff.
4. In your journal, jot down your first impression of the note. Make a note of what it smells like: fruity, nutty, spicy, etc. Take another sniff, a little more deeply and note your description. Exhale through your nostrils, and then inhale again to capture any notes or individual oils you may have missed in the earlier sniff.

5. Wait fifteen minutes and test again, inhaling your strips. Note any changes or additions you might want to make in your journal.

6. Wait another fifteen minutes, and take out a second perfume strip and write the essential oil name, time and date and "#2."

Top notes tend to evaporate rather quickly, losing their scent in 6-8 hours. Middle notes tend to last longer, 24-48 hours. Base notes remain the longest and do not dry out for many hours. They can last 48-72 hours.

7. Dip your perfume strip into the same essential oil as the first.

8. Now, take both perfume strips and compare the perfume strips, smelling the first one again.

9. Make notes regarding your impression of the body of perfume strip #1.

10. Focusing on blotter #2, revise your impression based on your comparison of both strips.

11. After half an hour (one hour since the first strip was dipped), smell strip #1 and make a concluding assessment of the body note. Compare to strip #2 for any differences in odor.

12. Continue to smell strip #1 at half-hour intervals to determine when the dry-out emerges. Write down your thoughts of the drydown and note how long it took for the scent to disappear completely. You might want even to wait and let them sit overnight to check again.

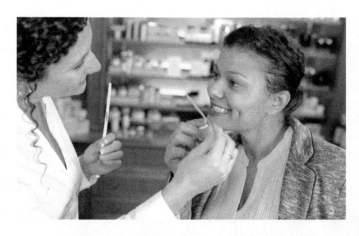

Be sure to refresh your palate from time to time so "olfactory fatigue" doesn't set in. After smelling too many scents, you may need to smell some coffee beans to clear your palate or take a deep breath into a wool scarf several times.

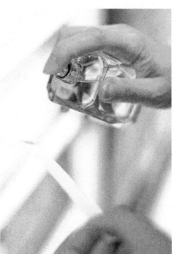

Once you start blending, you can get a preview of how a fragrance may smell by fanning multiple perfume strips in front of your nose.

HOW TO CORRECTLY SMELL AN OIL

When asked to smell something (hopefully something good), most people usually take a long, deep breath, dragging in the aroma. However, this is not the best way to smell an essential oil, according to some experts. Professional noses recommend taking a short sniff, then stop for a moment, then another short sniff, allowing the olfactory to retrieve the initial information gathered and to examine closer after each sniff. The nose will gather new information with each additional sniff. Three short sniffs should be taken, and then exhale. While the nose is capable of being able to distinguish over 10,000 odors, as a perfumer you will want to recognize each new scent, differentiate it and discover each's nuances, retain this new information, and commit it to memory.

The best time of day for working with new oils is later in the day when your palate is neutral rather than early morning. Make sure you are comfortable and relaxed during the process.

DESCRIBING YOUR FRAGRANCE

The perfume industry has developed its own language of scent borrowing many of its phrases from several other interests such as music and cooking in order to describe a fragrance. Many of these words have iconic meaning and are widely known. While there seems to be a consistent basis

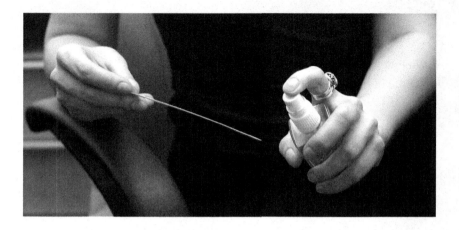

for perfume perception, being able to define your fragrance and convey its nuances is an important part of creating it. Developing a fragrance vocabulary will enable you to articulate similarities and differences with your customer, and they in turn will be able to share their preferences.

As you take the time to smell each essential oil, you will want to write down its fragrant characteristic and a description of its bouquet.

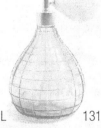

ODOR DESCRIPTORS

Below is a list of a few of the odor descriptors used in perfumery. Some of the terms listed may refer to their makeup or composition, while others describe their sensory perceptions or convey the physiological and psychological effects they have on humans. Complete the exercise by filling in the blanks with the name of an essential oil that fits each descriptive term as you become acquainted with their distinction.

Dry

Powdery

Fresh

Stimulating

Enlivening

Harsh

Crude

Imbalanced

Heavy

Light

Delicate

Musty

Rich

Sensual

Sharp

Penetrating

Sweet

Pleasurable

Soft

Delicate

Fragrant

Smooth

Sweet

Balsamic

Warm

Airy

Ambery

Bitter

Brisk

Floral

Cool

Citrus

Deep

Earthy

Euphoric

Light

Lemony

Leathery

Fruity

Herbaceous

Rancid

Rounded

Zesty

Masculine

Feminine

Musty

Nutty

Overbearing

Tart

Woody

Spicy

Sparkling

Soapy

Sour

Smoky

Medicinal

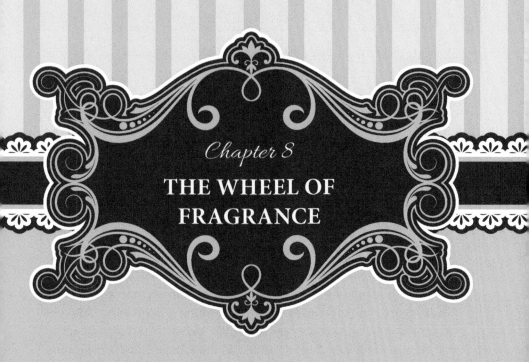

Chapter 8

THE WHEEL OF FRAGRANCE

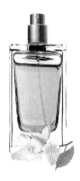

Sometimes a scent is more evocative than a photo or an image. It is a primer for the deflagration of sensation, emotions, desires, uncontrollable atmospheres, Deja vu that flood and wrap us like honey, until they make us drown in an unrepeatable moment of wellbeing... olfactory hallucinations that lead us anywhere: to the North of any South, to the East of any West...

– Profumum Roma

Essential oils are categorized into four major aromatic groups: Green/ Fresh, Floral, Oriental, and Woody. Within these four categories are fourteen families of aromas, according to scent expert Michael Edwards in his book *Fragrances of the World*. Edwards, a consultant in the fragrance industry, came up with a method for perfume classification showing the relationship between each individual fragrance family. His fragrance wheel, which is highly consistent with previous studies on odor descriptor and odor profile representations, shows how each family leads into the next. Those subcategories that fall under each major group consist of numerous combinations of fragrance notes, and because of this, a perfume made up of different notes and accords may fall in more than one fragrance category. As an example, Edwards explains, "Florals lead

*W*hen selecting essential oils for aromatic blends, you will want to select your essential oils from one or more aromatic groups based on their fragrance and odor intensity. Be sure to read each essential oil's profile and precautions to determine if it's the right match for your blends.

into soft florals when blended with sparkling aldehydes and balanced by a powdery drydown. Soft florals are transformed into floral orientals by adding the scents of orange blossom and sweet spices."

Since its creation, the fragrance wheel and its classifications have been modified several times with the addition of new aromatic groups to incorporate diverse fragrance types. Prior to 2010, the fougère aromatic family was placed in the center of the fragrance wheel, since its scents typically overlapped other fragrances from each of the other four main groups such as citrus from the Fresh family, oakmoss from the Woody family, coumarin from the Oriental family and lavender from the Floral family. [10]

Fragrance expert Laura Donna says, "These word groupings enable us to forge connections between perception and language. While they may be well known to diligent students of perfumery, other readers will relish new connections."

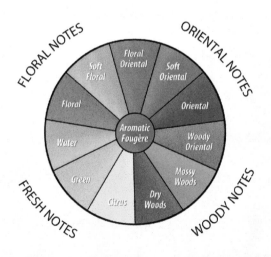

FRESH (Aromatic Fougère)

The Aromatic Fougère sits in the center of the wheel since its shares fragrances from each of the other families. Subgroups of Fresh Notes include **Citrus**, **Green**, **Fruity**, and **Water**. Traditionally, fougère's base comprises lavender, oakmoss, and coumarin giving it a sharp, woody scent. They are frequently used in men's fragrances.

FRESH (AROMATIC)

TOP (HEAD)	MIDDLE (HEART)	BOTTOM (BASE)
Anise	Allspice	Artemisia
Basil	Black Pepper	Benzoin
Bergamot	Cilantro	Ginger
Grapefruit	Clary Sage	Rosewood
Lemon	Lavender	Oakmoss
Lime	Nutmeg	Cedarwood
Mandarin	Peppermint	Jasmine
Orange	Sage	Patchouli
Tea Tree	Thyme	Rose
	Cannabis	Sandalwood
	Balsam Fir	Vanilla
	Cardamom	Vetiver
	Cinnamon	Tonka Bean
	Coriander	
	Clove Bud	
	Geranium	
	Juniper	
	Nag Champa	
	Rosemary	

FOUGÈRE

TOP (HEAD)	MIDDLE (HEART)	BOTTOM (BASE)
Bergamot	Allspice	Galbanum
Tea Tree	Cannabis	Jasmine
Grapefruit	Cilantro	Oakmoss
Lemon	Lavender	Rose
Lime	Balsam Fir	Sandalwood
Orange	Cardamom	Vetiver
Basil	Geranium	Tonka Bean
Lemongrass	Clary Sage	
Peppermint	Juniper	
	Sage	
	Pine	
	Thyme	
	Coriander	
	Lemongrass	
	Orris	

Citrus fruits offer a tangy and yet lively energetic spritz to fragrances. They are light and seem to perk you up! These provide a pleasurable tickle to the nostrils when used in fragrances. Citrus oils include bergamot, citronella, grapefruit, lemon, lemongrass, lime, mandarin, orange, tangerine, and verbena.

CITRUS

TOP (HEAD)	MIDDLE (HEART)	BOTTOM (BASE)
Anise	Basil	Artemisia
Bergamot	Cardamom	Ginger
Grapefruit	Eucalyptus	Oakmoss
Lemongrass	Melissa (Lemon Balm)	Patchouli
Lemon	Geranium	Rosewood
Lime	Juniper Berry	Sandalwood
Mandarin	Lemongrass	Vetiver
Orange	Neroli	
Verbena	Sage	
Tangerine	Thyme	
Tea Tree		
Petitgrain		
May Chang		
Citronella		

Green (Chypre) are fresh like a newly mown lawn, yet crisp and invigorating as a favorite perfume for men. The herbal scent brings out the natural, outdoorsy you! Perfumes made from this type are composed of essential oils such as cedarwood and pine with a twist of lime or lemon added. Other oils in this group include angelica root, basil, carrot seed, celery, clary sage, dill, fennel, hyssop, marjoram, rosemary, thyme, lavender, and juniper berry.

CHYPRE

TOP (HEAD)	MIDDLE (HEART)	BOTTOM (BASE)
Basil	Carrot Seed	Angelica Root
Bergamot	Clary Sage	Artemisia
Fennel	Dill	Cedarwood
Lemon	Geranium	Galbanum
Lime	Hyssop	Rose
Mandarin	Juniper	Benzoin
Orange	Lavender	Frankincense
Verbena	Marjoram	Labdanum
Anise	Pine	Myrrh
Tea Tree	Thyme	Oakmoss
Grapefruit	Rosemary	Rosewood
Lotus Flower	Violet	Sandalwood
	Eucalyptus	Patchouli
	Balsam Fir	Vetiver
	Cannabis	Tonka Bean
	Nag Champa	Vanilla
	Neroli	Ylang Ylang
	Peppermint	
	Sage	
	Verbena	
	Allspice	
	Black Pepper	
	Pimento	

GREEN

TOP (HEAD)	MIDDLE (HEART)	BOTTOM (BASE)
Eucalyptus	Clary Sage	Galbanum
Orange	Verbena	Artemisia
Anise	Balsam Fir	Benzoin
Coriander	Cannabis	Frankincense
Lemongrass	Cardamom	Labdanum
Peppermint	Cilantro	Oakmoss
Tea Tree	Juniper	Rosewood
Basil	Lavender	Sandalwood
Spearmint	Neroli	Cedarwood
Oregano	Rosemary	Vetiver
Bay Laurel	Sage	Helichrysum
Fennel	Pine	Calamus
	Thyme	Spikenard
	Chamomile	Valerian
	Juniper Berry	Tonka Bean
	Marjoram	
	Palmarosa	

Fruity compositions are made up of notes that are airy, fresh and invigorating; these are considered a favorite for summer. This group consists of various berries and citrus that are sweet and tart such as bergamot, lime, lemon, grapefruit, orange, and cinnamon.

FRUITY

TOP (HEAD)	MIDDLE (HEART)	BOTTOM (BASE)
Bergamot	Heliotrope	Violet
Grapefruit	Juniper	Vanilla
Lemon	Neroli	Ginger
Lime	Cinnamon	Jasmine
Mandarin	Carrot Seed	Benzoin
Orange	Roman Chamomile	Cedarwood
Lemongrass	Clove Bud	Oakmoss
Anise	Orris	Patchouli
		Sandalwood
		Vetiver
		Rose
		Ylang Ylang
		Rosewood

Water (Aquatic) includes bergamot, clary sage, cilantro, coriander, eucalyptus, jasmine, lemon, lemongrass, mandarin, sweet orange, peppermint, rose, rosewood, and verbena. Fruity and Water groups are mostly made up of synthetic oils.

WATER (AQUATIC)

TOP (HEAD)	MIDDLE (HEART)	BOTTOM (BASE)
Anise	Cilantro	Cedarwood
Basil	Clary Sage	Jasmine
Bergamot	Clove Bud	Oakmoss
Coriander	Geranium	Patchouli
Eucalyptus	Hyacinth	Rose
Lemon	Thyme	Rosewood
Lemongrass		Sandalwood
Mandarin		Vanilla
Neroli		Vetiver
Orange		
Peppermint		
Verbena		

FLORAL

The subgroups of Floral include Floral, Soft Floral, Floral Fruity and Floral Oriental.

Floral scents are classy, yet romantic. A bouquet of beautiful fragrances from this group will bring out the best in you! This perfume type includes feminine notes such as rose, jasmine, and ylang ylang.
Other oils in this group include Roman chamomile, German chamomile, geranium, lavender, neroli, and violet. **Soft Floral**'s main notes are aldehydes and powdery notes. **Floral Oriental** includes orange blossom and other sweet spices.

FLORAL

TOP (HEAD)	MIDDLE (HEART)	BOTTOM (BASE)
Anise	German Chamomile	Rose
Basil	Roman Chamomile	Jasmine
Bergamot	Clove Bud	Ylang Ylang
Eucalyptus	Lavender	Galbanum
Lemon	Geranium	Oakmoss
Neroli	Hyacinth	Patchouli
Orange	Thyme	Violet
Peppermint	Clary Sage	Cedarwood
Grapefruit	Heliotrope	Rosewood
Lemongrass	Juniper	Sandalwood
Acacia	Myrtle	Vanilla
Linden	Hyssop	Vetiver
Mandarin	otus Flower	Artemisia
Ambrette		Benzoin
		Ginger
		Labdanum

GOURMAND (FLORAL FRUITY)

TOP (HEAD)	MIDDLE (HEART)	BOTTOM (BASE)
Lemon	Allspice	Benzoin
Lime	Cardamom	Frankincense
Mandarin	Cinnamon	Ginger
Orange	Clove Bud	Myrrh
Anise	Nutmeg	Vanilla
Peppermint	Heliotrope	Tonka Bean
	Rosemary	
	Sage	
	Thyme	
	Nutmeg	
	Black Pepper	
	Pimento	

ORIENTAL

The subgroups of Oriental include Oriental, Soft Oriental, and Woody Oriental.

Oriental scents are exotic and sometimes sensual. This distinctive group of oriental notes leaves a waft of mystery behind. The perfumes from this classification are warm, long-lasting and tend to be on the heavy side. Fragrances for women often use a floral like jasmine or lavender, while men's fragrances use more of the earthy scents such as clary sage and citrus oils. Other oils in this group include palmarosa, frankincense, myrrh, vetiver, and ylang ylang, while sandalwood and patchouli fall in the **Woody Oriental** group. **Soft Oriental** includes incense and amber. **Spicy** scents are as comforting as mom's homemade apple pie, and allure you in an old-fashioned way. These groups of fragrant notes include bay, black pepper, cardamom, cinnamon, clove bud, coriander, ginger, juniper berry, and nutmeg.

ORIENTAL

TOP (HEAD)	MIDDLE (HEART)	BOTTOM (BASE)
Lemon	Lavender	Jasmine
Lime	Clary Sage	Palmarosa
Orange	Cinnamon	Frankincense
Grapefruit	Clove Bud	Myrrh
Mandarin	Bay	Vetiver
Coriander	Black Pepper	Ylang Ylang
Anise	Juniper Berry	Sandalwood
Bergamot	Cardamom	Patchouli
Fennel	Cilantro	Ginger
Bay Laurel	Neroli	Nutmeg
Lemongrass	Allspice	Artemisia
Lotus Flower	Verbena	Rose
	Geranium	Rosewood
	Heliotrope	Cedarwood
	Juniper	Labdanum
	Cassia	Benzoin
	Dill	Vanilla
	Cumin	
	Nag Champa	
	Nutmeg	
	Orris	

WOODY

Woody scents are deeply wooded forest notes that draw you in to explore yet deeper. This strong group of aromatic oils is worn by both men and women and is mostly made up of base notes of bark and moss. Perfumes made in this group include a woodsy, mossy and flowery accord. Essential oils that may be used in this perfume type include jasmine, rose, bergamot, cajeput, cedarwood, cypress, eucalyptus, myrtle, niaouli, petitgrain, pine, rosewood, sandalwood, tea tree, patchouli, and vetiver. **Mossy Woods** main notes include oakmoss and amber. **Dry Woods** main notes are dry woods and leather. **Oriental Woods** includes oils such as patchouli and sandalwood.

WOODY

TOP (HEAD)	MIDDLE (HEART)	BOTTOM (BASE)
Bergamot	Cypress	Jasmine
Cajeput	Myrtle	Rose
Eucalyptus	Niaouli	Cedarwood
Petitgrain	Pine	Rosewood
Tea Tree	Cilantro	Sandalwood
Basil	Cinnamon	Patchouli
Grapefruit	Clove Bud	Vetiver
Lemon	Lavender	Oakmoss
Mandarin	Neroli	Artemisia
Orange	Sage	Galbanum
Anise	Thyme	Ginger
Lemongrass	Allspice	Labdanum
Palo Santo	Balsam Fir	Benzoin
Ravensara	Cardamom	Agarwood
Birch	Geranium	Vanilla
Tulsi	Juniper	Opoponax
Neroli	Nutmeg	Peru Balsam
Lotus Flower	Black Pepper	Tonka Bean
	Spruce	
	Fir	
	Cannabis	
	Na Champa	
	Orris	

EARTHY

TOP (HEAD)	MIDDLE (HEART)	BOTTOM (BASE)
Basil	Thyme	Artemisia
Eucalyptus	Balsam Fir	Sandalwood
Orange	Cannabis	Benzoin
Peppermint	Cardamom	Frankincense
Anise	Cilantro	Galbanum
	Lavender	Ginger
	Black Pepper	Labdanum
	Rosemary	Myrrh
	Coriander	Oakmoss
		Cedarwood
		Patchouli
		Vetiver
		Opoponax

LEATHERY

TOP (HEAD)	MIDDLE (HEART)	BOTTOM (BASE)
Anise	Allspice	Artemisia
Tea Tree	Clary Sage	Benzoin
	Heliotrope	Galbanum
	Cinnamon	Vetiver
	Clove Bud	Frankincense
	Nutmeg	Labdanum
	Black Pepper	Myrrh
	Pimento	Oakmoss
	Pine	Rosewood
	Nag Champa	Sandalwood
		Patchouli
		Vanilla

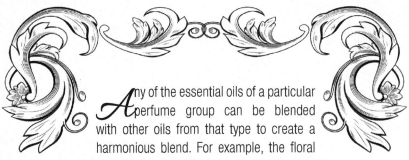

*A*ny of the essential oils of a particular perfume group can be blended with other oils from that type to create a harmonious blend. For example, the floral group can be blended with other oils from the floral group. The groups are arranged in a circle so that you can see at a glance each group and which essential oils are in that group.

Neighboring groups also blend well with the groups on either side. For example, geranium, a member of the floral group, blends well with orange, a member of the citrus group, or patchouli, a member of the Oriental group.

All groups can be mixed together, although some groups blend better than others. For instance, spicy and oriental oils blend well with floral and citrus oils; citrus, woody, and herbal oils blend well with green/herbal oils; and woody blends well with all categories.

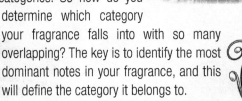

With so many perfumes on the store shelves, most experts classify fragrances into one of these main categories. So how do you determine which category your fragrance falls into with so many overlapping? The key is to identify the most dominant notes in your fragrance, and this will define the category it belongs to.

By identifying your personal favorites, you will learn about the fragrance families in perfumery. Consider each of the examples below and rate each one according to how strongly you like, dislike, or are indifferent to its scent.

Category	Scent	Like	Indifferent	Dislike
Musk, Oriental	Leather			
	Musk			
	Honey			
	Dairy cream			
	A burning candle			
Spicy, Woody, Bitter	Freshly cut timber			
	Church incense			
	Cinnamon			
	The earth after rain			
	Freshly cut grass			
Fresh, Green	A Christmas tree			
	Fresh strawberries			
	Mint leaves			
	Freshly washed linen			
	Lemons			
Floral	Baby powder			
	Magnolia blossoms			
	Lily of the Valley			
	Honeysuckle			
	Rose blossoms			

Did you find that most of the fragrances you strongly liked are in the same category? Commercial perfumes are usually based on one of these four fragrance categories. People are often drawn towards the same types of scents, so it helps to identify your preferences before you begin creating your own perfume.

Some people prefer the musky scents of the first category, which can be sexy, seductive, primitive and exotic. Sometimes overpowering, these fragrances are often more suited to the evening than daytime wear.

The spicy, woody, bitter family can be refreshing and invigorating. This includes fragrances such as sandalwood, cinnamon, vetiver, and myrrh. Masculine perfumes are often comprised of scents from this category.

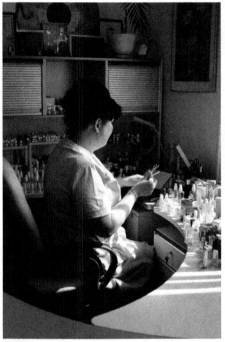

The third category represents fresh, green fragrances that are stimulating and awakening—such as clean, herbal scents like pine, eucalyptus, citrus, basil, rosemary, and lavender.

The floral category includes calming, soft scents—such as rose and jasmine—that are typically used in feminine perfumes.

Once you have identified your favorite fragrance family, you can begin experimenting with essential oils from that group. Try combining different oils from within the same family to create a blend that you find appealing.

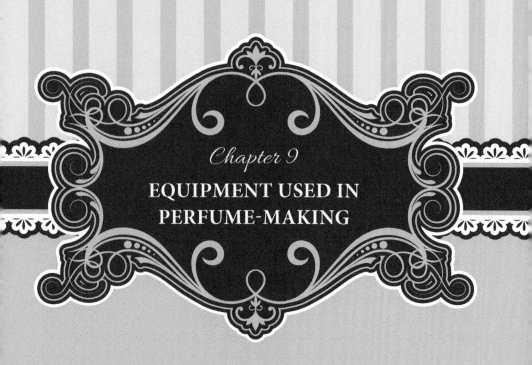

Chapter 9

EQUIPMENT USED IN
PERFUME-MAKING

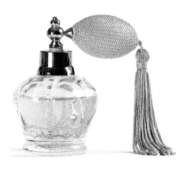

To create new arrangements, new olfactory forms, it is enough that you think "in odors," like the painter "in colors," and the musician "in sounds."

– EDMOND ROUDNITSKA

Having the necessary equipment available such as bottles, droppers, and containers will be a must before starting your perfume blend. Below is a list of the necessary tools you will need to get started.

EQUIPMENT

Glass Bottles in dark 5-milliliter, 10-milliliter, and 15-milliliter sizes with orifice reducers (plastic droppers) can be used to make topical essential oil blends. Standard bottles for storing your essential oils and accords can be purchased at SKS Bottle & Packaging.

Perfume Bottles such as decanters and small, delicately designed bottles for your perfumes can be purchased at flea markets, craft stores, and antique shops. The Internet offers many avenues for various shapes and size.

Plastic Bottles with a pump, squirt, or screw-off top are suitable for liquid soaps, shower gels, shampoos, lotions, and conditioners. You can find these in 2-ounce, 4-ounce, and 8-ounce sizes.

Plastic or Glass Spray Bottles are great to have on hand when making room sprays, facial spritzers or cleaning solutions. You will find these in 1-ounce, 2-ounce, 4-ounce, 8-ounce and 16-ounce sizes.

Small Glass or Plastic Tubs are perfect for bath salts, facial creams, salves, scrubs or other bath blends. These come in a variety of shapes and sizes from 2-ounce to 8-ounce.

Shot Glasses or Small Glass Bowls can be used for combining and blending essential oils. Have at least a half dozen on hand for different variations of an accord.

Plastic Transfer Pipettes come in different sizes and lengths for easy and precise drop measuring. They are ideal for filling small vials and for measure drops and small amounts of oils. Use these when you want to transfer oil from a large bottle into smaller bottles. They are for one-time use and should be thrown away to avoid cross-contamination.

Glass Eyedroppers are used to measure essentials oils during the initial stages of your perfume development. These allow you to use very small amounts and have more control over how much is used. Be sure to use the same size droppers for all the essences, so that you will be able to record accurate amounts when converting to weight in the future.

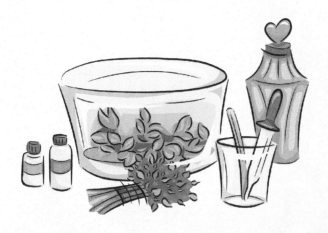

Clear Mini Atomizers are perfect for perfume samples. You can use these to make samples for friends and family to share (1-milliliter or 2-milliliter sizes work best).

Funnels are useful for pouring liquid from one container into another. Tiny brass funnels approximately 0.87 inches x 1.26 inches that hold about 3 milliliters of liquid are best for small containers. These and other perfume-making supplies can be found at Vetiver Aromatics.

Glass Graduated Cylinders or Beakers are made of thermally stable and chemically resistant borosilicate glass, so you don't have to be concerned about plastics corrupting your fragrances. Measurement lines start at 1 milliliter and demarcate every tenth milliliter. Using a cylinder for your formula allows you to form a true meniscus, facilitating accurate measurement.

Measuring Spoons will be needed when measuring larger amounts of liquids. Ordinary kitchen ones are fine for this purpose.

Rubbing Alcohol is good to have on hand for cleanup. You will need this for cleaning your glass droppers and utensils between uses. Never use isopropyl alcohol for creating perfumes, though. It is too strong and inappropriate for perfume-making.

Perfume Strips or Perfume Blotters are made for sampling an essential oil or fragrance. You will need these to test a scent, rather than just sniffing from the bottle. The strips will give you a more precise depiction of the smell and how it wafts. Using a perfume blotter strip allows you to experience the full range of your fragrance. These are strips of unscented, fairly stiff white absorbent paper that can be purchased online or you can make your own by cutting watercolor paper into ½-inch strips.

Scales, preferably digital, are great for accuracy in measuring your essences. A small, reliable set can be purchased online or at a craft supplies store locally.

Glass Stir Rods are great for stirring mixtures and make cleanup easy. You will also want to have toothpicks and/or bamboo sticks for blending as well.

Coffee Beans should be kept on hand in a small container for sniffing when your sense of smell has become weak. After sniffing several oils, you might lose touch and need to take in some deep breaths from the coffee tin.

Waterproof Labels are a must for labeling your bottles. You will want them in all shapes and sizes.

Perfumer's Journal or Recipe Cards are indispensable for keeping track of your formulas. You will want to write down the name of your perfume, the fragrance description, its ingredients, number of drops and more!

Traditional Japanese/Chinese Bamboo Earpicks are great for scooping out a drop of oil, such as a thick resin absolute that refuses to pour from the bottle. These bamboo picks have a tip on the end that curves up to hold a small amount of oil. These can be easily cleaned and reused.

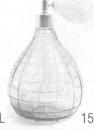

EQUIPMENT USED IN PERFUME-MAKING

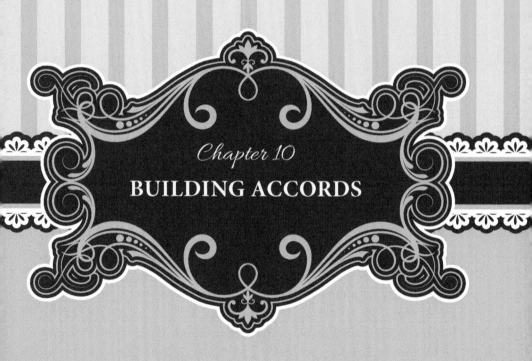

Chapter 10

BUILDING ACCORDS

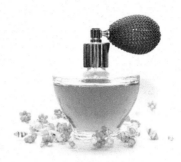

*I for one love perfumes that unveil themselves,
that one does not understand immediately; but
what is truly moving, what everyone is seeking,
is that scent which is closest to skin.
The reality of sensuality.*

– DOMINIQUE ROPION

How perfume is made seems to be shrouded in mystery. Professional noses remain tight-lipped and secretive, while the industry seems unwilling to share their techniques to a new world of inquisitive novice perfumers.

On the outset, it appears to be only mixing and matching essences, but as you will discover, it proves to be more of a balancing act between art and science.

Just as every painter approaches the blank canvas to begin his masterpiece with an image in mind, so does the perfumer in his or her approach to making perfume. Estée Lauder described in her autobiography *Estée: A Success Story* how she once smelled a green leaf at Palm Beach and instantly decided she must recreate the fragrance. "Aliage is sporty," Estée Lauder writes about her fragrance she described as "a woman walking onto the tennis court." Since she couldn't find a scent that emulated that feeling, she made one.

Whether one is inspired by a feeling, a situation, or even by nature itself, the rest of the process is hard work; as Thomas Edison said, "Genius is 1% inspiration and 99% perspiration." For Estée Lauder, nature inspired her to create an energetic, active sports spray that was a revolutionary concept at the time. What followed was hundreds of hours of hard work in bringing her vision to fruition—an idea that's still relevant today.

So, what does "sporty" smell like? And how does one go about finding the right combination of scents that would manifest and conjure up an image of "a woman walking onto the tennis court" when wearing it?

For professional noses, understanding chemistry is critical in deciphering the nuances of oils, the development, substantivity and reactivity of ingredients when making a fragrance. In 2011, there were over 3,000 materials used in scents for fine fragrances and consumer products. Of course, one perfumer may not be familiar with them all, but it's typical for an experienced perfumer to be aware of and have worked with hundreds of them.

As a beginner, it is not necessary for you to know chemistry (though it helps). It is, however, incredibly important to be familiar with the ingredients you use and dedicated to learning how to differentiate between their smells.

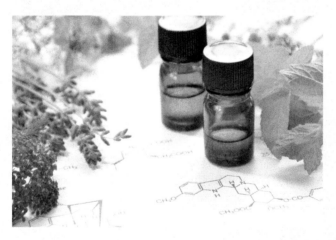

As you begin to familiarize yourself with your oils, you will notice some oils are intolerable undiluted and must be diluted at 10% or less to work with them. Some scents will be fleeting, while others will remain on the perfume strips for weeks. Other "still note" oils will need to be left out to air for a while before they are usable and you will find others that improve when aged. Some resinoids will need to be blended with a solvent (dipropylene glycol) before they are easy to work with. You may encounter oils that discolor the finished product, while others may react with each other to form new chemical compounds.

When it comes to blending with essential oil, you learn by experimenting and seeing what happens when you combine oil X with oil Y, and how to modify it to your liking. Mistakes, if you want to call them that, will train you in what throws a blend with an awful off-note. Discovering how to lift a fragrance and how to make it last will be significant, too.

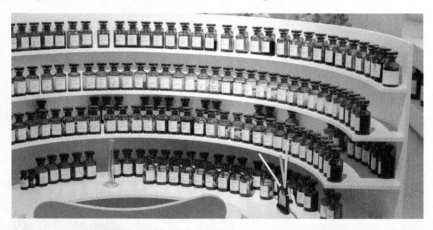

Spending time in front of the perfume organ making hundreds of adjustments and modifications to a single product will teach you these things. Ultimately it will be this working knowledge that will allow you to release your artistic flair in finding the ideal combination of oils that projects your vision and image to the wearer.

While the number of approaches to making perfume are as vast as the number of fragrances, as a self-taught perfumer, you will want to focus primarily on developing fine fragrances using some basic techniques, which means less emphasis will be placed on the technical knowledge. The good news is that once you understand the basic concepts, the rest is just hard work and practice.

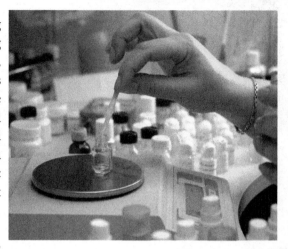

Systematic approaches used by traditionally trained perfumers in constructing a formula that helps a fragrance stick together and do what the perfumer intended it to do includes using accords. Creating and using harmonious accords as the building blocks for your perfume will allow you to create a fragrance that conveys your message just as Estée Lauder's legendary "Aliage" did in the 70s.

WHAT IS A PERFUME ACCORD?

A perfume accord is a combination of fragrance notes that collectively form the core structure or backbone of a perfume. Professional perfumers call it the "juice." Typically, an accord is made up of three to four notes containing a top, middle, and bottom note. In perfumery, accords are like chords in music—each is made up of different tones, but when blended together harmoniously form an entirely new scent, like a melody.

Considered an art as much as a science, an accord could also be compared to painting, such as when two colors are blended together like yellow and blue to create a new color: green. During the composition process of forming a blend, the notes lose their individual identity and create an entirely new odor impression. The key is creating something that can stand on its own and one in which you cannot detect its individual components. Many, many hours are spent on finding and creating the perfect marriage between scents since flawlessly made accords will be used again and again as a base from which other fragrances can sprout.

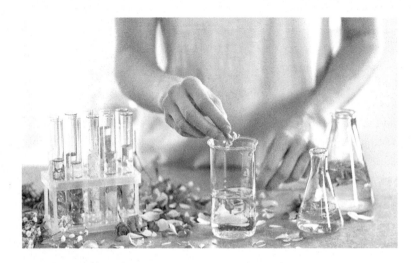

Add one or two notes to the accord and it will completely change the accord altogether and yield an entirely different perfume.

HOW TO CREATE AN ACCORD

The structure of an accord is like that of a pyramid with the base note being the largest part of your blend, approximately 30-55%. Even though this is the largest group of the total fragrance and tends to last the longest, it usually doesn't appear until after the "drydown." The middle notes make up 20-30% of your total blend, creating the heart of your fragrance. Top notes make up the smallest portion, approximately 15-40% of your fragrance.

You will find many variations in the percentages from different sources. For example, some experts suggest using a 40:30:30 ratio for the top, middle, and base notes respectively. Feel free to adjust your percentages as needed. In certain cases, it may be necessary to add more top or middle note when working with a heavier base oil so that they don't get lost in the blend.

BUILDING A VERTICAL ACCORD

As you begin, remember to follow your nose.

1. Take out all of the essential oils you want to use. Be sure to have a container of coffee beans nearby to smell between oils to clear your palate (nose). You will want to stop every few minutes to inhale the coffee beans or step outside for fresh air.

2. Decide on which medium you will be blending in, such as perfumer's alcohol or jojoba oil. Fill a 5 milliliter (1 teaspoon) bottle with it. It is recommended to work with oils at 10% dilution to get a better idea of what the final product will smell like. With this amount, you will be adding a total of 10 drops. For example, at a 40:30:30 ratio that would be:

   4 drops top note

   3 drops middle note

   3 drops base note

3. If you find the top note gets lost in the base oil and is not as outspoken as you would like, you can increase the number of top note drops and decrease the number of base note drops. For example, at a 60:30:10 ratio that would be:

   6 drops top note

   3 drops middle note

   1 drop base note

4. Choose 2-5 oils as possible choices for your chord. Use your perfume strips in deciding which combination of oils you want to use.

5. In each chord, one note will dominate, with the others supporting or enhancing it. You may start with your favorite oil, or choose oils from a favorite aromatic group. Select your dominant note first, then 2-3 oils that work well together.

6. Add each oil one drop at a time, smelling after each drop is added. Check your blend as it evolves and changes. Begin with one drop of oil (such as the base note) that smells strongest to you. After adding one drop of essential oil to your base oil, note what it smells like. This step is important in educating your nose as you learn to blend. All essential oils smell different once they are diluted.

7. Keep a notebook to list all of the oils in your accord. When you add a drop of essential oil, place a tick mark next to that oil's name.

8. Next, add the essential oil you have chosen as your middle note and pause to smell what these two oils are like together. Check how the two oils meld.

9. Continue with adding your top note and again pause to smell the new aroma.

10. Once you have added one drop of each note, you can begin to layer the blend by continuing to add different amounts of each oil.

11. Remember, you will want to balance the aroma of the blend. When blending several oils, you will be looking for specific characteristics for each of the different oils and those that will be strongest and dominant in your blend.

12. Once you reach your desired dilution and your blend smells perfect to you, you can stop. Be sure to write down your final number of drops (or count the tic marks in your notebook). Even if your percentage of drops for each note are not exact, it's okay. There are no hard and fast rules to structuring your composition.

Note: Stronger oils require fewer drops. Heavy oils such as florals (rose, jasmine, ylang ylang and geranium) can ruin a blend if too much is added. As you will soon discover, too many drops of certain oils may overwhelm your blend and even give you a headache. On the other hand, lighter oils, like the citruses, may require more.

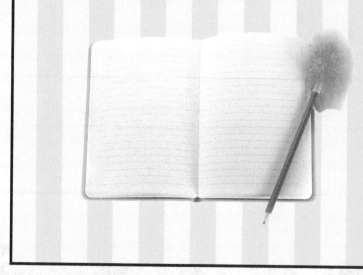

HORIZONTAL ACCORDS

A perfumer creates chords to use as building blocks in composing a blend. In a horizontal accord, only single notes of the same volatility rate are used—top note accords, middle note accords, and base note accords. Each chord will contain two or more notes combined together.

When creating your accords, you may want to choose oils from the same aromatic group that complement one another, or you may want to pick oils that contrast one another adding interest and flair to the chord. Here are a few examples of horizontal accords:

Top Note Accord

Floral - Neroli, Orange, Lemon

Middle Note Accord

Oriental - Cinnamon, Clove, Allspice

Base Note Accord

Leather - Frankincense, Myrrh, Sandalwood

After creating these accords, a perfumer can construct a fragrance using one top note accord, one middle note accord, and one base note accord, building layer upon layer. You may choose to use multiple chords to build a more complex blend, or only one chord such as a base note accord and then add single notes for your middle and top notes that will make a harmonious perfume. If you have several horizontal chords premade, you could possibly add a drop of each note for a more multifaceted formulation. A popular example of a base note accord is Amber, which contains benzoin, vanilla, and labdanum. For example, an Amber accord may contain:

5 drops Labdanum

4 drops Benzoin

1 drop Vanilla

Other accent notes such as clary sage, juniper berry or frankincense could be added to add mystery and differentiate the accord.

VERTICAL ACCORDS

When creating an olfactory impression, a vertical chord incorporates at least one note from each level of volatility rate—top, middle, and base. A perfumer can combine several vertical accords to create a multifaceted perfume. Or, a perfumer may choose one vertical accord to be the "central theme" of the blend, and add additional notes to create something new or different that complements it.

For example, the recipe below contains one top note, one middle note, and one bottom note following the simple 3-2-1 drop method:

Woody Accord

9 drops Basil (top note)

6 drops Cinnamon (middle note)

3 drops Vetiver (base note)

In this accord, all notes are members of the Woody aromatic group. When choosing oils for your vertical accords, you will want to look for ways each oil complements one another. Even if each oil is not from the same aromatic group, you may look for characteristics or other similarities that each oil shares or has in common such as invigorating (peppermint, rosemary, basil), or warm (ginger, black pepper, cinnamon).

A more systematic approach to creating a perfume accord is to take five shot glasses or small bowls and add varying amounts of drops of essential oils for comparison. In this example, we will be creating a top note horizontal accord that will create that immediate effect upon opening up your perfume bottle.

1. Take five shot glasses and number each glass using masking tape or labels and a marker.
2. Select the dominant essential oil for the chord you are creating. In this example, basil will be the dominant oil. Add your dominant oil to each shot glass starting with nine drops in shot glass #1, eight drops in shot glass #2, decreasing the number of drops in each glass to one drop in shot glass #5.
3. Next, choose the second, complementary oil for the accord. In this example, lime is used.
4. Add your second oil to each shot glass starting with one drop in shot glass #1, two drops in shot glass #2, three drops in the third glass, and so on, increasing the number of drops until each glass contains the number of drops as shown.

Shot Glass	#1	#2	#3	#4	#5 (number of drops)
Basil	9	8	7	6	5
Lime	1	2	3	4	5

5. Compare each glass by swirling and sniffing to determine which combination is the best one. The reason for not continuing with more than five drops of lime is that lime would then become the dominant oil.
6. Once you have selected the best ratio of oils, set that shot glass aside and move the other shot glasses away from your workspace. These will need to cleaned for the next step. For this example, shot glass #4 has been chosen. Our example blend contains six drops of basil and four drops of lime:

Shot Glass	#4
Basil	6
Lime	4

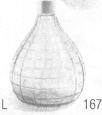

7. Now, take the third oil you have selected for this accord and add one drop at a time (between 1-5 drops) to this shot glass until you are satisfied with its fragrance.

    Note: Since, you are unable to take away drops once they have been added to a blend, you might want to continue with steps 8-10 and skip step 7.

8. Instead of using the drop-by-drop method in step 7, you can instead multiply the base formula by 5 in order to fill each shot glass for the next step.

    Basil 6 x 5 = 30 drops
    Lime 4 x 5 = 20 drops
    Total   = 50 drops

9. In this step, you will be repeating the process. Take five clean shot glasses that have been labeled #1 through #5 and add 10 drops of your oil blend to each glass. Continuing with our example we are adding the basil (6 drops) and lime (4 drops) combination to each shot glass:

Shot Glass	#1	#2	#3	#4	#5 (number of drops)
Basil/Lime	10	10	10	10	10

10. Now, with the third note you have selected for this accord, add the number of drops increasing in each shot glass. In this example, citronella has been selected.

Shot Glass	#1	#2	#3	#4	#5 (number of drops)
Basil/Lime	10	10	10	10	10
Citronella	1	2	3	4	5

11. Smell each shot glass and decide which one you like the best. If you chose to add additional oils to your accord, you will need to repeat the process each time.

With blending by note, you can create both vertical and horizontal accords as discussed earlier. However, the percentages of notes differ. Instead of using the ratio 40:30:30, you will follow the simple formula of using the 3-2-1 drop method. For every drop of the base note, you add 2 drops of middle note and 3 drops of top note. For example, an accord would look like:

WOODLANDS ACCORD
    3 drops Petitgrain (top note)
    2 drops Myrtle (middle note)
    1 drop Cedarwood (base note)

If you want to incorporate additional oils, you can use multiple oils for one note, keeping the ratios in proportion. In this example, two oils were selected as the top note, and two oils for the middle note:

    2 drops Petitgrain (top note)
    1 drop Lemon (top note)
    1 drop Myrtle (middle note)
    1 drop Juniper (middle note)
    1 drop Cedarwood (base note)

Using the blending by note method, you can create both vertical and horizontal accords.

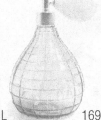

Choosing oils by aromatic group is another way to build a chord. Take, for instance, the following example. All three oils selected for this vertical chord are from the Oriental aromatic group.

ORANGE SPICE

    4 drops Sweet Orange (top note)
    3 drops Clove Bud (middle note)
    3 drops Ginger (bottom note)

It's totally up to you and your nose, so don't feel bound by the traditional methods. You, as the perfumer, can mix and match aromatic groups or methods in designing your formula. For example, in this accord, each note came from a different aromatic group.

FRUITY TOOTY

    4 drops Lemongrass (top note)
    3 drops Cinnamon (middle note)
    3 drops Vanilla (base note)

Lemongrass is from the Fruit group; cinnamon is from the Oriental group, and vanilla is from the Gourmand group. It's okay to think outside the box and combine essences from any group to create your accord.

THE MATRIX OF HORIZONTAL AND VERTICAL ACCORDS

As mentioned earlier, a note may consist of one or more accords creating a composition of multiple chords in a blend. For instance, your perfume might consist of three accords and look like this:

    4 drops Top Note Accord
    3 drops Middle Note Accord
    3 drops Base Note Accord

Or, you might use two drops of one top note accord and two drops of another top note accord. The combinations are plentiful.

Another interesting way to build your perfume is to start with one vertical accord (Oriental Accord) as your dominant accord. Then, choose a second, horizontal accord (Spice Accord) that shares the same heart note:

Top	Middle	Base
Orange	Cinnamon Clove Allspice	Ginger

You could do this using a base note accord or top note accord as well.

Top	Middle	Base
Lemon	Cinnamon	Benzoin
Orange	Clove	Ginger
Bergamot	Allspice	Patchouli

MAKING YOUR FIRST AROMATIC GROUP ACCORD

When blending aromatically, you will choose an aromatic group or groups to use first. From that group, you will select three or more essential oils for your accord. If you choose an aromatic group that does not contain all three notes, you may choose an oil from a neighboring aromatic group, or simply use only the oils from your group.

It may require a bit of experimentation with your essential oils to get the scent that you are looking for. Making an aromatic blend is definitely an art and, like any art, the result will depend on the time, inspiration and imagination that goes into the product.

You will want to analyze the various aroma groups to determine which ones you want to work with. Inhale each one and note your impressions. Build a file on each group and what the aromas of that group remind you of. Did you notice how they changed and developed over time? It's important to pay attention to how the fragrance makes you feel and how all of the oils you have chosen in a group will work together as a blend. What effects do you want to enhance? What distinctiveness do you want to emphasize and what characteristics do you want to tone down? Keep in mind to always strive for a balance in your choice of oils while maintaining their aromatic benefits.

The following chart is a sample recipe for each perfume type. Try one of these, or make up your own! Of course, perfumes are usually much more complex with additional oils, but this is a good place to start.

Aroma Group	TOP	MIDDLE	BASE
Citrus	Lemon	Neroli	Oakmoss
Floral	Petitgrain	Lavender	Jasmine
Oriental	Mandarin	Black Pepper	Ylang Ylang
Spicy	Orange	Nutmeg	Clove Bud
Woody	Basil	Cypress	Sandalwood
Herbal	Fir	Juniper Berry	Vetiver

Chapter 11

FIXATIVES

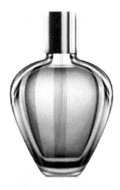

*There are no women who do not like perfume,
there are women who have not found their
scent.*

– Marilyn Monroe

I n times past, perfume odors were often made as infusions and not
distillations. This reduced the rapid loss of some of the odor quality
and characteristic of the plant. Perfume fragrances were once
expected to be quite tenacious, yet sweet while remaining elusive. This
led to the process of "fixing" scents, which entailed being able to select
odors that when blended with the most volatile components of the
perfume, prevented their rapid evaporation while still retaining the most
outstanding note of the fragrance. To achieve this, fixatives are employed.

Within this study of natural perfumery, fixatives are odorless and almost
colorless materials that slow down the rate of evaporation of the more
volatile materials in a perfume composition. This process gradually
causes a change in the scent of perfume as the ingredients slowly fade
away. Although fixatives may also lend a particular note to the perfume
throughout the stages of evaporation, it does not significantly affect the
evaporation rate of the other materials in the perfume. Fixatives are used
in fortifying, improving and stabilizing perfumes by paralyzing the odor
of the low-boiling (volatile) materials in the perfume.

FIXATIVES CAN BE CLASSIFIED INTO THREE TYPES:

Neutralize: these are chemical odors used in commercial perfumery

Agreeable: these are pleasant scents that harmonize such as benzoin, frankincense, tolu balsam, sandalwood, clary sage, and vanilla

Disagreeable: these are scents that may fortify or enhance, such as valerian, civet, Africa stone, castoreum, asafetida and jasmine

These fixatives will each slightly change the underlying scent of the perfume and modify them.

FIXING A SCENT

Fixatives slightly change the primary scent of a perfume by modifying it. There are three ways to fix a scent:

1. Adding fixatives to the alcohol (neutral or grain spirits) to complement the final perfume. Base alcohols that can be used include tonka bean or benzoin. Expert Jeanne Rose of "All Natural Beauty" states on her website, "The total amount of natural ingredient should be no more than 3 grams total per quart" (http://allnaturalbeauty.us/fixatives.htm). A 'fixative' must not necessarily be a part of the main scent.
2. Blend in scents that will harmonize with the primary odor you are trying to create.
3. Rosewood, mimosa, jasmine or tuberose can be added as final fixatives. Exalting fixatives, Rose says they are "the final fixative that improves or fortifies the main scent and are usually composed of animal notes that soften and smooth harsh notes." These should be included in trace amounts or small drops.

When studying the quality of the fixative or the tenacity of the oil, it is important to note that the two may not necessarily mean the same thing. While tenacity refers to the lasting effect of a perfume and its ability to linger on the skin, an aromatic perfume with regards to an ingredient may have immense tenacity but little impact on the evaporation rate or fixative qualities of the other fragrance ingredients it is combined with.

UNDERSTANDING THE LIMITATIONS OF FIXATIVES IN NATURAL PERFUMES

Keep in mind that synthetic perfumes differ from natural perfumes in terms of longevity (how long a perfume's fragrance lingers) and sillage (how it diffuses in the air when worn, leaving a trail behind). A botanical fixative may impart longevity and help prolong the sillage of a natural perfume; however, it may not be as effective as its synthetic counterpart. Although this may be a disadvantage or a determining factor to those who may want to choose perfumes made with aromatic botanical materials, perhaps what some consider as the ever-increasing assault of synthetic perfume ingredients on our olfactory organs have over time brought out a natural defense as the nose gradually became accustomed to these new scents. Natural/botanical perfumes offer users with alternatives and healthier options while still enjoying the benefits of a return to the much needed natural yet arrestingly beautiful scents of our world. Considering this, sillage and longevity is quite a small price to pay for one's comfort.

THE BENEFITS OF INCLUDING FIXATIVES IN NATURAL PERFUMES

Every day we are subjected to a multitude of smells, from the least pleasant to the most welcoming scent. For some people, natural perfumes are preferable as they bear no resemblance to the synthesized majority commonly displayed on the counters of our favorite department stores. This is because natural perfumes bear more semblances to the fragrances that in times past had all ingredients obtained either from plant or animal origin.

It is crucial to become familiar with and know the value of incorporating fixatives into perfume compositions to impart longevity. The smell of the perfume itself is a mixture of odors obtained from raw vegetables, such as fruits of flowers or from animal origins like the deer musk (musk) and the sperm whale (ambergris). However, animal fixatives, which were quite valuable in past perfume compositions, are now rare, costly or unavailable. There is also the question of it being illegal or unethical, and as a result, a lot of these formulations have been replaced by cheaper manufactured options. No matter the source, users can still enjoy a natural scent at a very low price.

AMBRETTE SEED

This fixative is known for its exalting effect and its high tenacity. It is distinctly floral with a characteristic smell of brandy or wine. It is often substituted for musk and blends well with rose, neroli, sandalwood, clary sage, cypress, patchouli, oriental and "complex" bases. Ambrette should be sparingly used.

VIOLET LEAF

When used in very low concentrations, violet leaf has fresh, green leaf odor with a floral undertone. The dry yet strong leafy scent with a hay-like undertone has great diffusion power. It also complements certain floral blends, such as hyacinth, muguet, and high-class chypres, and blends excellently with tuberose, clary sage, cumin, basil, most citrus oils, sandalwood, frankincense, lavender, rose and jasmine.

COGNAC

If you have ever perceived a sharp, fruity yet green herbaceous odor in a perfume, then chances are cognac was used as a fixative. It blends well with ambrette seed, bergamot, clary sage, coriander, galbanum, lavender, styrax, and ylang ylang. This is a somewhat oily liquid that has outstanding tenacity and great diffusive power. It should be used in trace amounts to exalt and give fresh, fruity natural notes.

FRANKINCENSE

Besides being a favorite Christmassy scent, this one also has a spicy odor that is warm and balsam-like. Its note is somewhat turpentine-like and should be used with very heavy fragrances. Frankincense blends well with basil, black pepper, bergamot, galbanum, geranium, grapefruit, lavender, orange, melissa, neroli, patchouli, vetiver, sandalwood, and other spice oils. It also enhances the sweetness of citrus blends in an intriguing way.

GALBANUM

Galbanum should be used very sparingly as it has a powerfully fresh yet extremely balsamic green leaf odor with a damp wood undertone. As a modifier, it blends well with lavender, oakmoss, fir, styrax, elemi, jasmine, frankincense, palmarosa, geranium, ginger, rose, verbena, ylang ylang, and oriental bases.

LIQUIDAMBAR (STYRAX)
Styrax is a very hard to find specialty oil with a pleasant and quite tenacious odor. It works well as a fixative with a distinct aroma that enhances ylang ylang, rose, lavender, carnation, violet, cassie and spice oils.

VETIVER
Vetiver has a deep, earthy, woody scent with a sweet and persistent undertone; it can be used in oriental bouquets, and with frankincense, patchouli, oakmoss, sandalwood, violet, ylang ylang, galbanum, geranium, jasmine, lavender, clary sage, cassie, and rose.

MYRRH
A popular choice as an excellent fixative with a smoky, warm, sweet balsamic odor, myrrh also has a medicinal odor but blends excellently with violet, white rose, and lavender. It also blends well with frankincense, sandalwood, oakmoss, cypress, juniper, mandarin, geranium, patchouli, thyme, mints, and spice oils, and is used in heavy floral blends.

OAKMOSS
Oakmoss has a very broad, general usage as it is used to give perfumes of all kinds a natural undertone. It has a rich, earthy, bark-like odor. It has a high tenacious and fixative value and blends well with virtually all other oils, including lavender and ylang ylang.

ORRIS ROOT
Sweet, delicate orris root has a floral-woody odor. It blends well with carnation, cassie, cedarwood, bergamot, vetiver, cypress, geranium, mimosa, labdanum, clary sage, rose, violet, and other florals.

PATCHOULI
It has a strong, pungent, and earthy-herbal odor that is frequently used in oriental bouquets. Other oils that go well with patchouli include bergamot, black pepper, cassie, cedarwood, cinnamon, clary sage, clove,

elemi, frankincense, galbanum, geranium, ginger, jasmine, labdanum, lavender, lemongrass, myrrh, neroli, oakmoss, orris, rose, rosewood, sandalwood, and vetiver.

SANDALWOOD
An excellent fixative for vanilla, sandalwood has a soft but deep sweet-woody balsamic fragrance. It blends well with violet note perfumes, bergamot, black pepper, cassie, clove, geranium, jasmine, labdanum, lavender, myrrh, oakmoss, patchouli, rose, rosewood, tuberose, and vetiver.

VANILLA
Vanilla is perhaps one of the most universally known and favorite scents. With its unsurpassed richness, it supplies depth to many types of sweet-floral or heavy amber bases and oriental perfumes. Vanilla also blends excellently with sandalwood, vetiver, balsams, and spice oils, lavandin and lavender.

AMYRIS
Amyris mildly blends with various essential oils such as lavandin, oakmoss, citronella, rose, and Virginian cedarwood.

ANGELICA ROOT
This should be used quite sparingly as it has unique tenacity and a great diffusion power. It blends well with patchouli, oakmoss, clary sage, vetiver, and unique citrus blends.

BALSAM OF PERU
Balsam of Peru is an excellent fixative for heliotrope, rose, magnolia, and lilac perfumes.

CEDARWOOD, ATLAS
With its woody-balsamic odor and warm camphor-like top note, it blends well with bergamot, cypress, cassie, clary sage, jasmine, frankincense, juniper, labdanum, lavandin, neroli, rose, rosemary, vetiver, ylang ylang, oriental and floral bases.

CISTUS LABDANUM

Cistus has a characteristic ambergris-like odor, as well as a herbal-balsamic and leathery fragrance. It blends well with oakmoss, clary sage, juniper, lavender, lavandin, bergamot, cypress, vetiver, sandalwood, patchouli, frankincense (olibanum), and oriental bases.

CLARY SAGE

With a herbal-sweet, nut-like fragrance and an unusual tenacity, clary sage is somewhat reminiscent of tobacco, ambergris, sweet hay, and tea leaves. It is an excellent fixative that can be used with perfumes of a more delicate bouquet, and with bergamot, cedarwood, citronella, cognac, cypress, geranium, frankincense, grapefruit, jasmine, juniper, labdanum, lavender, lime, and sandalwood.

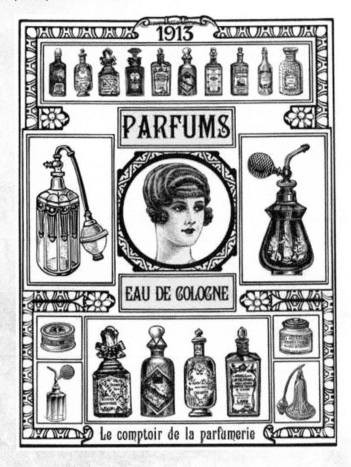

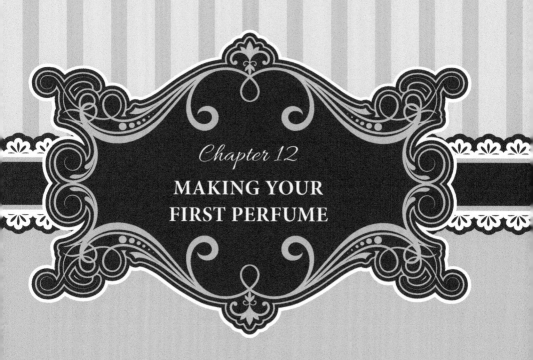

Chapter 12

MAKING YOUR
FIRST PERFUME

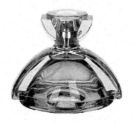

When I was a boy, I thought scent was contained in dewdrops on flowers and if I got up very early in the morning, I could collect it and make perfume.

– OSCAR DE LA RENTA

Now that you have learned about notes and accords to use in your perfume, it's time to make your first perfume.

1. Before you begin, gather all of the necessary equipment: bottles, pipettes, essential oils, paper towels, labels, vials, and/or containers.
2. Make sure the counter space is clean, and the area you are working in is well ventilated. You may want to put down wax paper (or a paper towel) to prevent any damage to the countertop from accidental spills. This will also make cleanup much easier.
3. If you haven't already done so, formulate three accords for your top note, middle note, and base note. To do this, choose and combine oils that form a harmonious blend. Make sure no particular oil stands out unless you have chosen one to be dominant, providing the main identity of your accord.
4. Inhale the fragrance. If this fragrance is not what you had in mind for your perfume, choose another accord and test again. Once you have chosen the accords or oils for your perfume, fan out all the perfume strips and wave them beneath your nose to see if you like it.

5. Start with your heart accord (middle note) first and work on finding a base note accord that complements it. Next, choose your top note that complements the other two accords. Check by using your perfume strips with a drop of each accord on it. Hold beneath your nose and sniff. Once you are satisfied with your selections, you can blend.

6. Fill a 5-milliliter bottle or small glass bowl with one teaspoon of alcohol or jojoba oil*. Using a pipette, extract each accord into the bottle (or bowl). Remember to use a separate pipette or glass eyedropper for each of the oils used.

7. To create a sample using a 40:30:30 ratio at 10% concentration, you will be using a total of 10 drops in a 5-milliliter container. Begin by adding 3 drops of the base accord and mix well. Next, add 3 drops of the middle accord, checking the scent after each drop making sure it "marries" well with the base. Feel free to use less or more as needed. Continue by adding 4 drops of the top accord, adding a drop at a time and checking the scent each time. Be careful to add one drop at a time. One drop too many can alter the results. Replace the cap on the bottle and shake to mix oils together.

8. Once you are finished, consider what your modifier will be, if any. Also, consider if you want to add an accessory note, etc. Use sparingly.

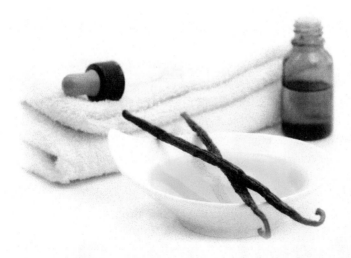

9. Allow the sample to sit for 24-48 hours to cure. Check your blend again to review final results.
   - Has the top note dissipated or disappeared? (You may need to add more top note.)
   - Has the middle note lost its identity? (You may need to add more middle note.)
   - Has the base note become too distinct during the drydown? (You may need to use less base note.)
   - Has the modifier or accessory note become too apparent? (You might want to change or disregard the modifier.)
   - If necessary, made adjustments and check the blend in 48 hours. If you find the fragrance pleasing to you, allow additional time for the fragrance to settle and see if the oils work together harmoniously, or cause discord.
10. Once you are happy with your sample, you can redo your formula at the higher concentrations and accords undiluted based on the type of product you are making.
11. Add your essential oil blend to a carrier (alcohol, water, lotion, gel, etc.) in the bottle or container and mix well to distribute the oils. What you use as your carrier and how much to add will depend on which method of application (Spray, Cologne, Perfume, etc.) you chose.

*If jojoba base oil is used, you may want to add more top note to compensate the heaviest of the oil.

READY, SET, BLEND

1. Have a notebook and pencil handy to write down the formula. Write down how many drops of each accord or essential oil you use, so you will know the final formula of your blend and can duplicate it later. (Trust me, you will forget how many drops you used of each oil if you don't do this!)
2. Have coffee grounds on hand to sniff between fragrances to help clear your palate.
3. Use a clean glass dropper or disposable pipette for measuring individual oils. Never use the same dropper for different oils as this will cross-contaminate the oils.

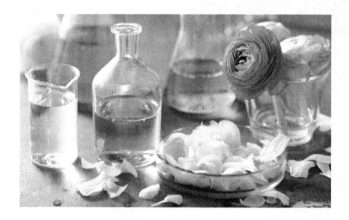

4. Never measure or mix essential oils with plastic utensils since the plastic will hold the scent of the oils. Some oils like cinnamon, clove bud, and orange will actually dissolve the plastic. Glass or metal works best for measuring.

5. Select your blending method and/or type of product you want to make. The aim is to create a blend that is perfectly balanced, without any overpowering individual scents. The synergy of aromas together should form a perfume that is more beautiful than its component parts.

   Tip: Since essential oils are potent in their purest form, you may want to dilute them to a 10% dilution when experimenting with them. Once you are happy with the results, then you can blend with them in their potent form.

6. Shake well to mix and then let it set for a day to allow the blend to breathe.

7. Add a label to your bottle with your blend name, date, and ingredients.

FOUR CONSIDERATIONS THAT WILL AFFECT THE FINAL OUTCOME OF YOUR PERFUME

- The type of carrier used for delivering the essences such as alcohol, jojoba oil, or beeswax.
- The percentage (or concentration) of essential oils used in the base or medium.
- The ratio of essential oils for the top, middle, and base notes.
- The delivery application chosen (spray, dab, etc.).

What is your favorite perfume? We all have our own preferences when it comes to scents that we find appealing. This is due to a complex combination of human biology and psychology. The human nose contains around 400 olfactory receptors, each of which can interpret a smell differently from person to person. So, while one person may find the smell of sandalwood pleasant, another may find it repulsive.

Also, our past experiences of scents can influence our psychological reaction to a particular smell. The olfactory bulb is linked with the limbic system of the brain, which is associated with memory. This is why a whiff of a certain fragrance can instantly recall a specific memory associated with that scent, whether it reminds you of a particular person, place, or period of time. A negative past association with tea tree, for example, may cause your brain to find this scent off-putting in the future.

Every perfume is comprised of a particular combination of aromatic compounds. It is possible to recreate a close approximation of your favorite perfume by identifying its unique ingredients and then blending the relevant essential oils. You may not achieve an exact copy, but the

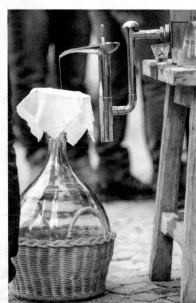

resulting scent should be similar to the original.

The beauty of making your own perfume is that you can create a blend that is completely unique and tailored to suit your individual aromatic preferences.

HOW DO I START?

The first step is to identify the key components of your favorite perfume. Using an online fragrance database, such as Fragrantica.com, is an easy way to research the notes contained in thousands of commercial perfumes.

As an example, I have chosen the popular men's fragrance Joop! Homme:

Perfume	Joop! Homme
Top Notes	Orange Blossom, Mandarin Orange, Bergamot, Amalfi Lemon
Middle Notes	Cinnamon, Cardamom, Lily of the Valley, Heliotrope, Jasmine
Base Notes	Vanilla, Patchouli, Tonka Bean, Sandalwood

Fragrantica also provides a useful list of notes that were identified by reviewers, in order of the number of votes received. For Joop! Homme, the results were:

Notes	No. of Votes
Vanilla	391
Cinnamon	382
Heliotrope	310
Tonka Bean	276
Jasmine	223
Sandalwood	207
Orange Blossom	201
Patchouli	172
Cardamom	139
Mandarin Orange	88
Lily of the Valley	88
Bergamot	77
Amalfi Lemon	45

This shows that the majority of reviewers identified vanilla as the strongest component in the perfume, followed by cinnamon. Some scents are easier to identify than others, so it is perhaps not surprising that the familiar scent of vanilla ranked more highly than the lesser-known tonka bean, for example. These results also illustrate the huge variations that result in smell perception among people who test any given perfume.

BLENDING

By experimenting with these key ingredients, you should be able to blend a perfume that has a similar scent to Joop! Homme. You will need to experiment with different ratios of these notes to find the perfect combination. Some scents are much more overpowering than others, and therefore will only require a minuscule amount. When dealing with essential oils, sometimes only one drop is all that is needed.

A perfume will usually contain around 15-40% essential oil, while a lighter eau de toilette may only have a 5-8% concentration.

As a base for your perfume, you can use fractionated coconut oil or perfumer's alcohol. If you cannot source all the fragrance notes, try to find suitable alternatives—for example, it will be easier to obtain regular lemon essential oil, rather than amalfi lemon.

Once you have discovered a balanced blend of notes, store the perfume in a dark-colored glass bottle away from heat and light.

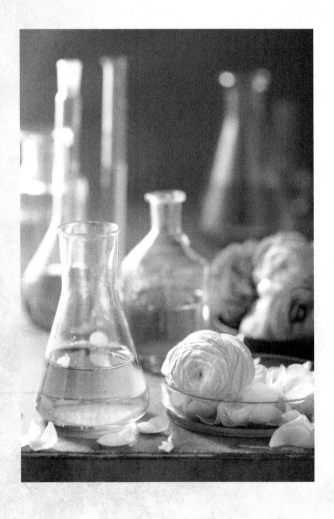

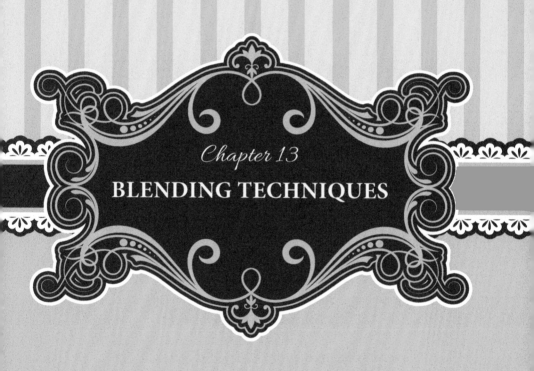

Chapter 13

BLENDING TECHNIQUES

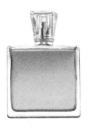

Perfume is ... 'that last and best reserve of the past, the one which when all out tears have run dry, can make us cry again.'

– MARCEL PROUST, NOVELIST

In choosing a particular essential oil to start with, consider its note and what other oils blend well with it. You will want to look at the fragrance wheel for ideas, or the Companion Chart on page ___ for suggestions.

Many perfumers start with the middle note(s) of what they want to use. Since this is considered the "heart" of your blend, decide what you are trying to achieve and what type of product your blend will be used in. Ask yourself these questions:

> *What is the purpose of my perfume?*
> *What is the mood I want to create?*
> *What are the age groups and/or sexes I am targeting?*

Next, choose your complementary base note(s). You will want to use your perfume strips to see how they smell together. Lightly fan the strips with the middle note(s) and the base(s) notes together beneath your nose and sniff to determine if they go well nicely together.

Finally, to finish off your blend, add complementary top notes(s). In some cases, you may want to use a modifier or bridge note in your blend at this point.

WHAT IS A MODIFIER?

A modifier can be added at the end to offer your fragrance its uniqueness or add a twist to it. These should be used sparingly. It is recommended to start with just a drop and increase slowly. Add a drop, then smell. If you can smell the modifier, then you have added too much. If this happens, increase your heart note. Don't forget to jot down each time you add a drop. You will want to keep a record of your recipe for future reference.

WHAT IS A BRIDGE NOTE?

A bridge note is a single note whose scent is used to connect two notes of a fragrance, smoothing out the transition from one phase to the next. Some perfumers recommend using this fourth note to help the other oils blend together. A bridge note, for example, may be lavender, peppermint, chamomile, marjoram or vanilla.

WHAT IS A FIXATIVE?

Fixatives are oils that bind various fragrances together, whether it's single notes or chords. A fixative can be any natural substance that will hold and "fix" the fragrance longer on the skin. In the perfume industry, this is a crucial element since most alcohol-based scents are fleeting and you need something to anchor the scent, thus lowering the evaporation rate.

Some of the more popular fixatives include myrrh, cistus labdanum, frankincense, balsam Peru, patchouli, spikenard, ylang ylang, vanilla, and sandalwood essential oils. Orris root and benzoin are both excellent fixatives but are sensitizers, which must be taken into consideration when used. Vitamin E oil, jojoba oil or another carrier oil can be used.

As you can see from the examples listed here, most fixatives are bottom (base) notes and aromatically can significantly impact your fragrance. For this reason, many believe these should be kept to a minimum. However, many of these can be integrated into your blend as part of your base and play an important part of your formula by retaining the predominating note of the fragrance.

Because of their strong scent, fixatives are usually kept to a minimum of 3-5% in a perfume. These usually consist of 0.2-0.5% of the final product.

Scents such as myrrh, spikenard and marjoram are good for women's perfumes, and frankincense, patchouli, and sandalwood are good for men's fragrances. Hopefully, you will be able to find a fixative that is agreeable with your blend and will work in harmony with the primary odor you are trying to create. Ginger essential oil adds spice and warmth, while oakmoss and vetiver work well with herbal or woody scents. Other fixatives that can bridge your scents well include rose, rosewood or jasmine for their sweet floral fragrances.

HOW TO TELL IF YOUR BLEND IS BALANCED

A well-composed blend will smell like one fragrance. You should not be able to detect any individual note or different parts. Your perfume will develop and change over time as it ages, but in the end, it will be considered either woody, soft and floral, spicy, fruity, etc. The fragrance will evolve revealing the top, middle, and bottom notes respectively over time, but it should not change from one scent to another to yet another during this time.

REACTION IMPACT

Certain essential oils have a greater impact and potency, if you will, especially when blended with other oils. For example, geranium can be an overpowering scent, whereas chamomile has a much softer and subtle

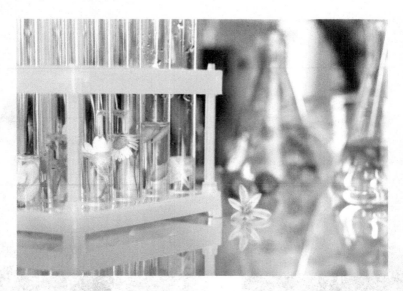

fragrance. If you use the same number of drops of each, the chamomile gets lost. Reaction impact is learning how to balance your oils so that they will enhance and complement each other in your fragrance.

DRYDOWN PERIOD

When a perfume is designed, it is created most importantly with the drydown in mind. This is the lingering scent of the base notes and how they react with the wearer's innate scent to make an individual effect. The top or head notes are the first to evaporate, followed by the middle or heart notes. The drydown in all takes around 30 minutes to elapse and what is left behind is an entirely original scent—that of the fixatives and base notes mingled with the chemistry of one's skin.

While the basis of the scent is the same in everyone's bottle, it is an extraordinary phenomenon that the aroma will suit one person differently from another. Considering how elusive a factor it is, a good drydown the sign of the work of an incredibly skilled blender.

One of the key differences you will discover with using all-natural ingredients such as essential oils and absolutes is that their evolution to drydown on the skin is unique to the materials chosen, revealing the true characteristics of the aromatics. Unlike some perfumes that contain synthetics, there isn't a "one note" linear scent from the first application to drydown.

TESTING YOUR SCENT

Although you may like two different fragrances, don't assume that they'll make a good mixture of perfume. First, test your possible blend on tester strips, so you won't waste your essential oils on combinations that don't work.

HOW MANY INGREDIENTS SHOULD MY PERFUME HAVE?

The number of ingredients a perfumer may use in a composition ranges from twenty to one hundred, but of these, only about six to nine define the fragrance. Other fragrances used in minuscule amounts balance, harmonize and decorate the fragrance.

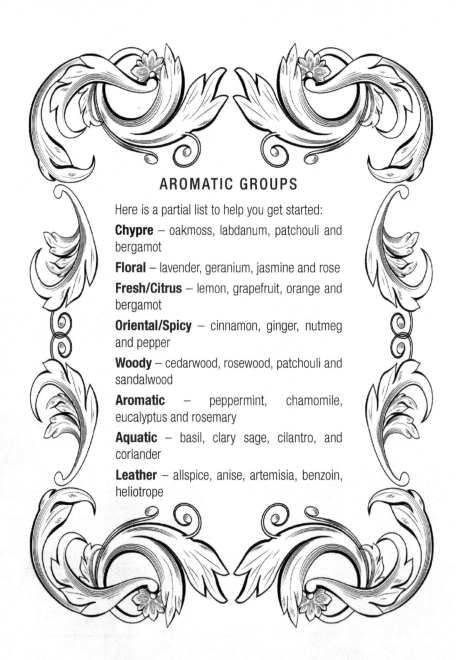

AROMATIC GROUPS

Here is a partial list to help you get started:

Chypre – oakmoss, labdanum, patchouli and bergamot

Floral – lavender, geranium, jasmine and rose

Fresh/Citrus – lemon, grapefruit, orange and bergamot

Oriental/Spicy – cinnamon, ginger, nutmeg and pepper

Woody – cedarwood, rosewood, patchouli and sandalwood

Aromatic – peppermint, chamomile, eucalyptus and rosemary

Aquatic – basil, clary sage, cilantro, and coriander

Leather – allspice, anise, artemisia, benzoin, heliotrope

The great perfumer, Francois Coty, created very simple formulas, yet his fragrances set the perfume world on its ear. It wasn't because of the number of ingredients he used. What was amazing was what he was able to accomplish using only a handful of ingredients.

As a natural perfumer, you might only use a few ingredients to start with. What's important isn't how many ingredients you use, but rather how the notes communicate with one another. Modern day fragrances tend to have fewer ingredients, giving the creator more control over the quality and availability of components. You can make your blend much richer in scent and pleasantly unique by adding more oils.

SUBSTITUTING INGREDIENTS IN A RECIPE

You will find a vast array of oils to choose from when creating a perfume. However, with over 200 types of essential oils, absolutes, resins, CO2 extracts and carrier oils available, purchasing every essential oil on the market could become rather expensive. This is why knowing how to substitute an essential oil in a recipe with another essential oil can enable you to be able to choose from the groups or scents you already have on hand and slowly grow your collection of essential oils gradually as budget allows. Naturally, your blend may vary slightly in aroma from the original recipe, but in many cases, the outcome will produce comparable results.

Here are a few things to take into consideration:

* The aromatic characteristics of the original oil and its substitution.
* The blending nature of the oil that will replace the original oil.
* The purity and quality of the oil that will replace the original oil.

When substituting essential oils in a perfume, your primary focus will be on the essential oils' aroma. In some cases, the essential oils you use in your blend may have a very different smell, but this is acceptable as long as the aroma is still agreeable to you.

It is best to replace essential oils from the same family or group—Floral, Citrus, Spicy, Woody, and Herbal. See Chapter 8, The Wheel of Fragrance for a complete list of essential oils for each group. Having a working knowledge of these basic groups is an easy way to remember which oils complement each other and serve as great substitutes in your blends.

Naturally, when blending essential oils with fragrance in mind, you should always follow your nose. There will be essential oils that blend well together and complement each other and others that won't. Be sure to check the profile for each essential oil you have in mind to see if it makes an excellent companion with your other oils before starting your blend. See **Appendix C: Companion Oil Chart** for more information.

Let's say, for example, you are using a recipe that calls for rose otto, but you don't have it on hand. You could try substituting rose geranium or another floral in its place. Although the two oils will not produce the exact aromas, the results of these two florals will be very similar. You can also try using rosewood instead.

If you are creating a blend that calls for cinnamon bark essential oil and you only have cassia on hand, try using it. Both of these essential oils are so similar in fragrance they are easily mistaken for the other.

Citrus oils such as sweet orange, mandarin, and tangerine are very similar as well and can be substituted for one another.

In much the same way, you can substitute and replace neroli oil, jasmine oil, and ylang ylang oil. Though all three are different from each other in

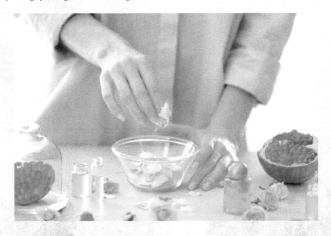

WHY DO SOME PERFUMES HAVE COLOR?

Natural perfumes, like their synthetic counterparts, can have color too. Essential oils may be brightly colored, depending on the flower or botanical it comes from. When working with these essential oils, perfumes will take on their hue.

Depending on which oils you choose, you might enjoy using essential oils that are attractively hued that will tint your perfume in a jewel-like style. If you like experimenting with color, here are some oils to consider when adding visual drama to your fragrance:

Amber – Bay Rum, Benzoin, Tuberose, Champa, Cinnamon Leaf, Myrrh

Brown – Tobacco, Balsam, Vanilla, Cistus Ladanum, Spinach Leaf Absolute

Golden Brown – Cassia, Ginger, Myrtle, Sandalwood, Valerian, Calamus

Dark Blue – Blue Tansy, German Chamomile

Green – Green Tea, Cumin, Clary Sage, Geranium Absolute, Oakmoss, Osmanthus, Verbena, Violet Leaf, Vetiver, Yarrow

Light Green – Carnation Absolute

Turquoise – Lavender Absolute

Orange – Carrot Seed, Boronia, Orange, Tagetes, Pink Grapefruit, Mandarin

Red – Rose Absolute, Jasmine Absolute, Lotus Pink Absolute, Patchouli

Yellow – Lemon, Lemongrass, Lime, Ylang Ylang, Allspice, Cedarwood Atlas, Roman Chamomile, Cinnamon Bark, Geranium, Pennyroyal, Tangerine, Tea Tree, Tuberose Absolute

Pale Yellow – Amyris, Cardamom, Celery Seed, Clove Bud, Citronella, Dill Weed, Palmarosa, Fennel, Hyssop, Juniper Berry, Lemon Myrtle, Litsea Cubea, Marjoram, Oregano, Peru Balsam, Ravensara, Lotus White Absolute

Clear – Aniseed, Anise Star, Basil, Bay Laurel, Bergamot, Birch, Black Pepper, Cajeput, Cedarwood Virginian, Coriander, Cypress, Eucalyptus, Fir Needle, Frankincense, Lavender, Lavandin, Galbanum, Helichrysum, Niaouli, Nutmeg, Peppermint, Petitgrain, Pine Needle, Rosemary, Rosewood, Sage, Spearmint, Spruce, Wintergreen

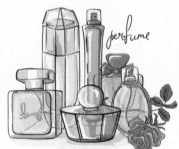

almost every way and have a distinct yet exotic aroma all their own, you can find these work as substitutes for one another. Another suggestion for substituting neroli is to use equal parts of mandarin, orange, and petitgrain to reach the required amount. So if the recipe calls for 4 drops of neroli, use 2 drops of mandarin and 2 drops of petitgrain instead.

Tea tree is commonly called for in recipes. However, if you should happen to run out, you can use equal parts of cajeput and lavender to achieve the desired amount.

Equal parts of cajeput and petitgrain can be substituted for melissa, which may be a bit hard to find.

Lavender is an essential oil you should never be without, but just in case you are in a pinch and don't have any on hand, try using chamomile instead.

Sandalwood essential oil is one of the most well known aphrodisiacs in the world and can be pretty pricey. As a substitute, you could use benzoin and cedarwood in equal parts.

If you don't have bergamot, try using grapefruit instead. Clary sage is used for balance in blends for both men and women, but if you're out, use sage and nutmeg in equal parts.

Some more common substitutions include:

Lavendin and Lavender
Grapefruit and Lemon
Clove Bud and Cinnamon
Spearmint and Peppermint
Jasmine and Neroli
Ylang Ylang and Cananga
Sweet Orange and Tangerine
Vanilla and Benzoin

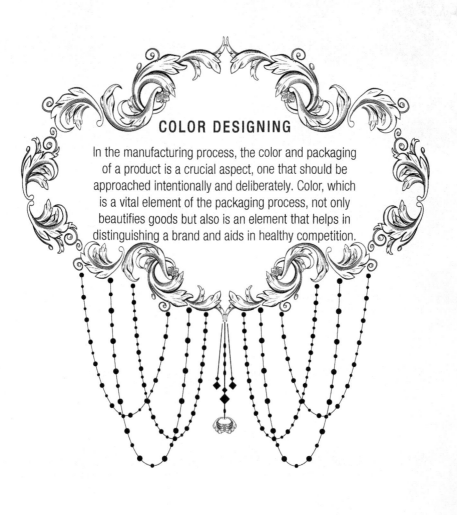

COLOR DESIGNING

In the manufacturing process, the color and packaging of a product is a crucial aspect, one that should be approached intentionally and deliberately. Color, which is a vital element of the packaging process, not only beautifies goods but also is an element that helps in distinguishing a brand and aids in healthy competition.

COLOR IN PERFUME

Novice perfumers may worry about their perfume's color. No doubt, you will notice certain essential oils add a tinge of color to your blend. This may or may not have any bearing on the final outcome of the product, but is worth taking into consideration when making body creams, for instance. Why not try to intensify the distinct look of your product with sparkling color?

WHAT DOES THE COLOR OF FRAGRANCE AND PACKAGING SUGGEST?

Sometimes, it is all about the packaging, especially the choice of color, when marketing a new product or an already existing one and fragrances are not left out in this rule. Sometimes, the color of the bottle or the box is not entirely unrelated to what it smells like. Most popular fragrances that have gained acceptance over the world employ this strategy when packaging their products. For instance, Bvlgari Aqua for men comes in a pebble-smooth, round bottle of the color of aqua to suggest an "aquatic" fragrance; Encre Noire by Lalique has the similitude of an ink pot in India and its scent is accordingly inky.

A GAME OF COLORS

The strategic link between fragrance and color is an old and proven one. Most of the time, the color of both content and container attempts to strike a balance, taking into consideration the theme or the chosen name of that particular fragrance. Chanel, for instance, is known for its mark of stark austerity, which promotes elegance in refusal and also the beauty of being different. In the words of its founder, Gabrielle "Coco" Chanel, Chanel fragrances began so as to make women "not smell like a flower bed."

Sometimes, the color of the fragrance is a play on the mind, and this stems from the fact that certain schools of thought and indeed design researchers assume that it is possible to establish a relationship between the senses of vision and smell. For instance, when one thinks of freshly cut grass, the color that comes to mind may most likely be the color a manufacturer may use to brand his or her own scent. Most times, before even sniffing the tester bottle on the counter, one almost certainly knows

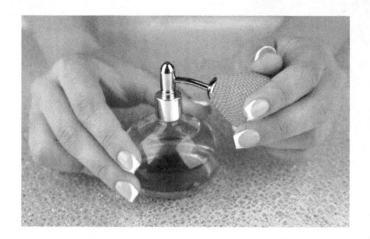

what to expect. It should also be worthy to note that most contemporary fragrances are not only transparent but also dyed with specific skin-safe dye that gives them an attractive hue customers tend to love so much.

Packaged fragrances mostly search for a line of divide, especially when there has to be a distinguishing factor for a male or female scent. Women are largely drawn to sweet-smelling and fruit-like odors and generally would also go with the girly colors, pink, lilac or orange, when choosing a fragrance color. A typical example is Prada's Pink Candy.

A blue packaging like Cool Water by Davidoff often suggests scents that are manlier and herbal-like. They are what one would call classic scents for men and are most times reminiscent of a beach smell or sea notes.

Purple, though glamorous, suggests a more unisex fragrance as the color tends to appeal to both sexes. However, sometimes it could be still girly but glamorous at the same time. Poison by Dior is a typical example of a purple scent.

For packaging that may be inspired by nature, the color green is most times chosen as it indicates freshness or tells of a romantic smell. Believe by Britney Spears or Guerlain Homme are examples of this.

Although "black" in a fragrance might make a powerful statement, it is very uncommon to find such fragrances on the counter as customers most times shy away from buying those due to fear of stains. However, there are a number of choices such as Jasmin Noir by Bvlgari or Lady Gaga, which dries clear.

White packaging most times signifies purity and a sense of peace and well-being. Most white packaging come in transparent bottles and fragrances and tells a story of pleasure and attraction. An example of such is CK One, which was a huge trend in the 1990s.

Red, which was earlier mentioned, most times suggests to the mind a hot, sexy or erotic scent. A typical example is Heat by Beyoncé, which not only depicts the voluptuous singer but tells of the sexy, warm scent contained in the bottle.

Manufacturers may also be inspired by nature's flora and fauna, especially flowers. One such flower is the rose. Packaging can intentionally predict the presence of a rose smell depending on the name or color of the fragrance. Dolce & Gabanna's Rose The One and Givenchy's Very Irresistible are typical examples of perfumes inspired by roses.

ARE THESE RULES UNCHANGING?

These rules are never binding and are always subject to change; there will always be exceptions due to customer preference or trends. However, it is advisable to flow with the tide; strawberries or peach packaging for the gentlemen may not be the best choice!

Based on the "7-Second Law," which suggests that a consumer at the point of purchase will make the decision whether to purchase a product or not in seven seconds, it is important to note that potential customers of a particular product are first attracted by the packaging and then the content. In those seven precious seconds of decisiveness, color accounts for about 67% of the determinant factors of "color marketing." Most perfume manufacturing companies use this to market their product.

Fragrance is not only an important part of everyday life but almost a necessity we cannot live without. After all, who would want to smell like hydrogen sulphide or ammonia when there are a lot of sweet-smelling options like vanilla and jasmine? Every individual wants to be associated with a particular fragrance or smell. There are a whole lot of different perfumes, and each comes with its own color. A particular color distinguishes one fragrance from another and most times stands for one character trait or individual personality. Blue, for instance, represents loyalty and truth. For the outdoor-loving individual, it may mean "sea" or "refreshing." Blue is most times assumed to be a masculine color, and most women who opt for that tend to be the freedom-loving or tranquil ones. Take Davidoff's Cool Water, for example—it not only allows users to feel refreshed like the feeling after a day at the beach, but can also be used by the ladies in summer.

The color purple is associated with royalty and as such when used for a particular fragrance gives an elegant, gorgeous and arresting impression. For women who desire or have an elegant and mature temperament, purple is the best option for them.

Pink comes in different shades, and as it is typically associated with women, it gives a gentle, lovely, shy and romantic impression. The fruity smell that accompanies most pink fragrances can brighten up a room full of people and go a long way in helping to meet new friends.

Yellow perfume gives people a luxuriant, downy, exalted, worshipful and a little bit sexy feeling together with a healthy dose of mystery. For the person who has a social status to live up to, this choice is most suitable for them to show their taste. An example of a perfect yellow fragrance is Chanel No. 5.

Givenchy's Greenergy perfume that comes in a light green color is a remake of nature, and it sedates the atmosphere around consumers. Green represents new life and is milder than blue. This product sends out a completely relaxed and comfortable smell and is perfect for women who lead a stressful life and want to create a peaceful and quiet environment.

Color design is important to every business as it attracts target customers. It also simplifies the advertising process for the manufacturers as a customer would automatically pick a product that best fit their person and by so doing cut cost. Improve your business and meet different customer needs by producing the desired colored perfume.

When creating a perfume, you'll inevitably come across an essential oil that doesn't want to budge from its bottle. While most essential oils feature a thin, almost water-like consistency, others such as absolutes or resins that have a much thicker consistency make it nearly impossible to pour, measure in drops or blend with other oils. For instance, myrrh (*Commiphora myrrha*), which comes from a gum resin, has a very thick consistency, while benzoin (*Styrax benzoin*) becomes almost solid at room temperature.

Most people choose to heat their oils in order to get them to a more workable consistency, but care must be taken to heat the oil gently and briefly, so not to potentially destroy some of the oil's constituents. One of the safest methods for loosening up thick oils is to gently warm the bottle in a water bath.

Follow these simple steps when using the water bath method:

1. Fill a small bowl with warm water. The water should be warm enough to affect the temperature of the oil, but not boiling. Loosen the cap on the bottle, allowing the contents to expand, but make sure water cannot get inside the container.

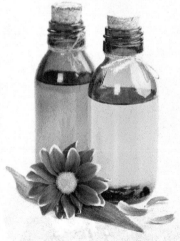

2. Place the jar or small bottle of oil inside the warm water. Allow it to sit for 10 minutes or until the oil is at the right consistency to work with. Different oils will vary in how much time it takes to liquefy.

3. If the water becomes cold within this time, replace it with warm water.

Tip: If your bottle label is not waterproof, place clear tape over the label to protect it before submerging into water.

The water bath method not only works great for essential oils, but also works well for absolutes, balsams, and resins such as benzoin and cistus labdanum. Keep in mind that different oils will take varying amounts of time to liquefy depending on its type, how solid it is and its ability to soften.

If you are planning on using a carrier oil in your blend, be sure to heat the carrier oil as well. This way, the oils will smooth out more evenly when mixed together. Most absolutes dilute more quickly in alcohol than carrier oil.

MEASURING THICK OILS

Measuring out your thick oil by the drop, even after it has been warmed, can be sometimes difficult to calculate. The aromatherapy standard for drops is 20 drops per milliliter of essential oil, depending on the viscosity of the oil. For instance, the thicker the essential oil, the fewer the drops per milliliter and vice versa; the thinner the oil the more the drops per milliliter.

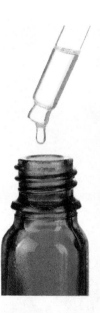

Most regular-sized aromatherapy pipettes are designed to give you approximately 20-25 drops per milliliter. Thicker oils like patchouli and sandalwood have the tendency to produce larger drops, while thinner oils such as lemon and orange produce smaller drops and drip off more quickly. Since most aromatherapy recipes designate drops, they are typically using the 20-25 drops as the milliliter standard.

You may find it beneficial to purchase disposable pipettes that are marked for each milliliter so that you can accurately measure the correct amount of oil needed for your recipe; otherwise, you may end up "guesstimating" what constituents a drop and counting one at a time.

Once you have calculated the number of drops per milliliter for a particular essential oil, write it down. This way you will have this information ready for future blends. Also, when creating your blend, you will always want to try to use the same style or type of dropper, so that your recipes come out consistent.

For blending small quantities, using the dropper method works well.

For larger amounts, measuring by milliliter works best. Some perfumers prefer to use digital pocket scales to weigh out the thick oil in fractions of a gram.

*A*s a perfumer, you will want to measure your ingredients in weight (ideally using a scale in order to work with precise measures). This will be important if you plan on duplicating a formula and/or making in larger quantities. For instance, some essential oils are thick and viscous like Cistus ladanifer or Onycha (Benzoin), while others are thin like Frankincense or Grapefruit that pours out quickly. A 15-ml bottle of an essential oil may contain the same amount in terms of mass, but by weight may differ. For instance, Frankincense will weigh less than one drop of Cistus ladanifer. You will want to use a scale to give you a formula's precise weight.

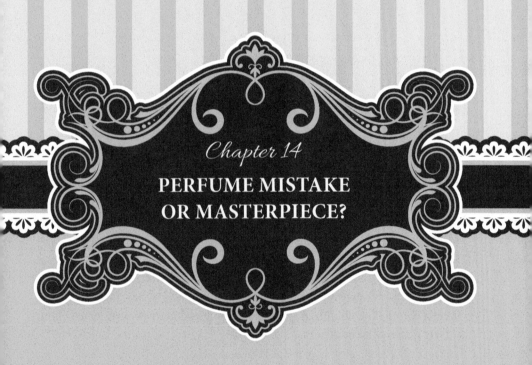

Chapter 14

PERFUME MISTAKE
OR MASTERPIECE?

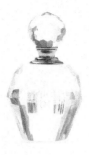

Aiming to balance too much a perfume, one turns it off, killing in it everything giving its character. There's no need to fear nor to avoid a dominant in a perfume... this "fault" has often been at the base of a great success.

– JEAN CARLES,
LEGENDARY TWENTIETH CENTURY PERFUMER

To try to list all the common mistakes people make when they make perfume is a bit like describing why the Mona Lisa turned out badly. Some of the greatest scents in the world have been made manifest by an overly zealous hand or an incorrectly chosen bottle.

Indeed, Ernest Beaux, the genius creator of Chanel No. 5, was quoted saying, "When I use vanilla, I make crème anglaise; when Jacques uses vanilla, he makes Shalimar." One person's translation of a note will be utterly different to another's.

Often fragrance disasters happen as a person tries to emulate another's work. They have not studied the nuances of the note well enough, sensed how it opens out and listened to interplay with the other ingredients. One's person symphony, when played by another perfumer, lacks life, imagination and harmony.

One of the main mistakes that leads to these disasters is people do not spend enough time measuring the reaction impacts of each note. Does it shout over the top of the others or does it whisper sweet nothings in the background?

Another is taking the time to understand the balance between the notes. Loving the floral accord or placing too much emphasis on the heart or head note can cause the scent to have a disappointing drydown, lacking in the fixative qualities of the base vibrations.

It stands to reason the more ingredients you have at your disposal, the more diverse your experimentation can be. Over time you will find that while you may have disregarded celery seed as a rather flat top note, blended with other accords it can make a blend sing. Notes such as vetiver with the sensuous weight can take on an almost angelic timbre when combined with the right harmony and in the right amount. Don't write off an ingredient simply because it does not please your nose…it may be you have not yet witnessed its whole picture.

The biggest mistake people make is trying to create a recipe in a linear fashion. They write a recipe down and then charge into pouring ingredients into a bottle. This is not only literally a recipe for disaster, but a very costly one at that!

Choosing three or four magical notes whose notes chime in blissful harmony allows you to discover a rough-edged diamond. Any others you add should merely polish the jewel.

By far the biggest tip I can give you here is to use your perfume strips as your first step. Don't be in a rush to add droplets of oil to your bottle. Layer the papers together, and it will be easier to add and take away notes and rectify perfumery mistakes in your formula as you go.

ADDING FRAGRANCE TO YOUR PRODUCTS

You may experience unexpected results when you add fragrance to your product. Some reactions that may appear include a change in the look and consistency of your product.

Because fragrances are primarily essential oil-based and many formulas are water-based, a non-ionic solubilizing surfactant such as polysorbate 20 or 80 may be used. Add your fragrance to the surfactant before adding to the final product. The amount of solubilizer needed will vary from product to product. A general rule is to use three to four times the amount of solubilizer to fragrance.

Adding fragrance to a product may make it thinner, especially in shampoos and body washes. When this happens, you might want to add a pinch of salt to the final product after the fragrance has been added. Be sure to test your blend in a small amount of base before making larger amounts. This is a process of trial and error, and results will vary.

Some fragrances may change the appearance of your product (especially clear gels) and cause them to look cloudy, hazy or even yellow. They can also cause the emulsion to separate or go grainy. This is why it is important to test your product's stability, especially if you are planning on reselling your products to the public.

Be sure to add your fragrance at the end of the formulation process. Adding your formula too early while the product is still warm could cause negative consequences. The more volatile components of the fragrance could evaporate off if still hot. This could also cause the fragrance not to smell as expected. If heating is not required, the fragrance can be added during the oil phase of your formula.

When creating a product line, you may want to use the same fragrance in different products. However, a fragrance used in shampoo may not smell the same as in a body lotion or cream. One solution may be to adjust the percentages in the fragrance to cover variations in the base odor. Be careful not to overcompensate, though, as the fragrance formula may also cause varying reactions when applied to the skin.

IS THE PRODUCT STABLE?

It is important to perform stability testing since you will be working with natural fragrances that contain many reactive groups. Testing should include storage under conditions of high heat. This will allow you to see

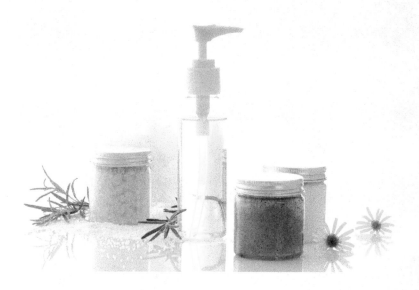

how increased heat may drive potential reactions that may change the scent and color of a product. One possible solution to help with heat stability is to add an antioxidant to your products such as Vitamin E. The antioxidants in Vitamin E can react with the free radicals to neutralize their ability to react.

Intense lighting is another factor to consider and should be tested. Exposure to light may turn a formula yellow or make it smell foul. When considering packaging, the type of plastic the product will be stored in will be paramount as it can also change the odor of the product. PET plastic is one type of plastic that may be used with fragrance. In cases where the fragrance is sensitive to light, dark-colored packaging should be used.

COMMON MISTAKES IN PERFUME-MAKING

When you decide to begin making perfume, it is a delicate art, to say the least. Humans are all different, and while one person may love the smell of lavender, another may detest it. Also, you need to make sure that you use the right amount of perfume. Otherwise, you could choke out the air, and that pleasant smell will become overpowering. Rather than relieve stress, you may only increase it.

Here are some of the common mistakes with perfume-making that you should be aware of to avoid.

MIXING TOO MUCH

When people first start to make their own perfume for aromatherapy, one of the biggest mistakes is that they simply mix too much. It can be expensive to make aromatherapy perfumes, and making a huge seven-ounce bottle is just too much. You can get by with making one cup of perfume and working with that. Another reason this is a big mistake is that if you made a large batch that didn't turn out right, that is a costly mistake of resources.

NOT LETTING IT CURE

A longer infusion may or may not always translate into something smelling better. Sometimes, after you have made all of your adjustments, you will find that two or more components don't work well together and cause discord, which ends up ruining your fragrance. Allowing the blend to sit for 48 hours and longer may in certain cases cause the oils to settle into harmony. However, sometimes the blend will simply be a failure that you will have to find another use for. But don't fret or worry, you are training yourself on what doesn't work. If further adjustments are made, you will want to allow it to sit for several more days. Who knows—maybe the next time will be the sure hit!

POOR STORAGE

It is important that you store your perfumes properly. For starters, you want to make sure that your perfume is stored in a small, air-tight container. You don't want to let air into that container, nor allow your infusion to get out. That is just a waste of great aromatherapy. You should keep it in a location that is room temperature, and not subject to temperature swings (a cold or hot room). Changing temperatures can cause the container to expand and contract, which will allow the perfume to leak in and out.

RUSHING

In your quest to make a perfume, you may want to rush things to get it done quickly. Aromatherapy is a science, and a balance must be found to create the right scent. If you rush things, you can ruin an entire batch and waste hours of your time.

When you get started making your first perfume, set aside a time when you can relax. Choose the oils you want to include and begin to mix them sparingly. By being mindful of these mistakes beginners often make, you are starting off on the right foot.

FAQ AND TROUBLESHOOTING

1. *Why does my perfume blend only last a short amount of time?*
   This is often due to the blend not having a harmony to the chord. In other words, consider the balance you have between the head, heart and base notes. The head notes, being very volatile, should disappear quickly, ushering in the heart notes and then leaving behind the weight of the base notes.

2. *My perfume is too strong. Can I dilute my perfume?*
   Adding a blend of nine parts alcohol to one part distilled water will dilute the blend without impairing the structure.

3. *How long should I leave my fragrance to sit?*
   As long as your patience will allow, and then a bit longer! Leave the blend for a week to see how the notes work together before you dilute. When you are happy, add your alcohol mix and then leave for 4-6 weeks.

4. *Are natural oils better than synthetic?*
   Not necessarily; they are simply different. In fact, in some ways, the synthetic versions may have the edge as the note can be adapted to bring out the exact nuance the perfumer wishes to exalt.

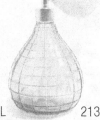

5. *How many drops should I use?*
   The viscosity of the oil will determine this, as the thicker the oil, the larger the drop. Myrrh oil, for instance, has a thick treacley consistency, whereas head notes such as lemon are thin. A general rule of thumb for calculating the number of drops is 600 to make one ounce of oil or 100 for a teaspoonful.

   As a perfumer, you will use the materials you need to achieve the exact effect that is desired—no more, no less. To err in either direction will weaken the effect of the fragrance. The art as a nose is in knowing when to add one more drop and when to leave it out.

6. *Why has my perfume gone cloudy?*
   This is usually due to some kind of contaminant, often a water droplet. Keeping perfume in a cool, dark place can avoid condensation building inside of the bottle, which is usually the problem.

7. *What packaging keeps perfume longer?*
   Perfume stored in a spray bottle works best. Atomizers reduce the amount of contact the blends can come into with the air.

8. *My solid perfume won't harden. What should I do?*
   You may have added too much oil and not enough beeswax. Try reheating the product and adding more beeswax.

9. *My perfume turned cloudy when I added hydrosol. What did I do wrong?*
   Add less hydrosol (or water) next time and make sure you are using perfumer's alcohol that is designed for colognes.

10. *My perfume feels sticky on my skin. How can I keep this from happening?*
    You might want to adjust the concentration of oils used.

Chapter 15

TYPES OF FRAGRANCES

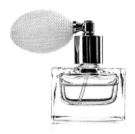

Oil and perfume bring joy to the heart.

– PSALM 27:9

While choosing a perfume may seem daunting enough with the differences between scents, compounds, and application methods, it is made all the more difficult when discovering the different varieties of perfumes. The types of perfumes include perfume or extrait, eau de parfum, eau de toilette, eau de cologne, and eau de fraiche. The most noticeable difference in all of these products is the different concentrations of essential oils that they possess. These differing strengths lend different properties to each product, affecting longevity, scent, and strength.

PERFUME

Perfume, also called extrait or extract, is the strongest of all the varieties, but certainly not the most common. Perfume can contain fifteen to forty percent perfume concentrate, also referred to as essential oil concentration or juice. This high percentage of essential oils means several things for the user. The perfume requires less to be applied to reach the desired effect, and the fragrance will last longer. When considering the percentage of essential oils in a product, it is important to remember that the higher the perfume concentration, the lower the amount of alcohol in the product—although alcohol is always present. Alcohol allows the fragrance to dissipate so others can smell it. This type of fragrance commonly lasts up to six hours and is the product quoted when testers and researchers state a good perfume will last six to eight hours. However, this increase in concentrate also means it usually costs more. **The length of time on the skin:** all day.

EAU DE PARFUM

Eau de parfum is the next strongest, behind extrait. Eau de parfum contains eight to fifteen percent perfume concentrate and is touted to last for three to five hours. It is a lighter perfume, with a lighter, easier-to-handle scent. For daytime or office use, this one would usually be preferred and is advisable to select over perfume simply for the fact that perfume, with its high concentration, can have the tendency to overpower other scents and give some people a headache with its strong smell. Eau de parfum, sometimes converted to the acronym EDF, is also cheaper than extrait. **The length of time on the skin:** almost all day.

EAU DE TOILETTE

Eau de toilette is the next strongest, behind both extrait and eau de parfum. Eau de toilette can also be expressed as EDT. Eau de toilette will have a much weaker concentration of perfume concentrate than extrait, having only four to eight percent concentration of the essence. Eau de toilette is even cheaper than eau de parfum, again due to its decrease in concentrate. Eau de toilette is probably the easiest product to wear on a day-to-day basis and has a very little possibility of overpowering anyone. It is said to last for two to four hours, making it an on-the-go perfume. This is a more popular perfume type because it is cheap and replaces the stronger perfume in many ways. **The length of time on the skin:** 80% will have evaporated in 4-6 hours.

Top notes:
The scents that are perceived immediately on application of a perfume

Middle notes:
The scent of a perfume that emerges just prior to when the top notes dissipate

Base notes:
The scent of a perfume that appears approx. 30 minutes after departure of the middle notes

EAU DE COLOGNE

Eau de cologne is the next to the weakest of the four options, with a perfume concentrate percentage of only three to five percent. With its low concentrate, it only lasts for about two hours. Eau de cologne can also commonly be referred to as ECF, or just cologne. A modern version of eau de cologne is known as eau de fraiche. **The length of time on the skin:** half an hour, with remnants of it after 2-4 hours.

Eau de fraiche is considered a cologne body splash with a very low concentration of perfume. It is the most affordable fragrance but must be applied several times a day due to its short-lived nature.

The different types of perfumes account for different percentages of alcohol. Being composed of animal and plant-based esters, the concentration of scented particles to the amount of solvent determines the category that the product falls into, i.e. whether it is a cologne, eau de perfume, eau de toilette, or perfume. **The length of time on the skin:** 90% will evaporate within 4-6 hours.

THE DIFFERENCE BETWEEN PERFUME AND COLOGNE

A common belief among society is that cologne is for men and perfume is for women, which is simply not the case. The easiest discernible difference that can be made between colognes and perfumes is that colognes have a weaker, more subtle scent. Other differences lie in how the scent is created, how it is perceived, and its potency. The ingredients that a company selects to make either perfume or cologne are different as well, which is what helps them to have different scents associated with them and also leads to the stigma of cologne being a male-only tool and perfume being only for ladies. The word "cologne" originates from Cologne, Germany and originally had a citrus base. The word "perfume" originated in France and was popular in the sixteenth century when Crusaders returned to the Middle East with their spoils from Europe.

A perfume consists of three scents that are also known as layers of the fragrance. It possesses a top note, middle note, and bottom note. The top

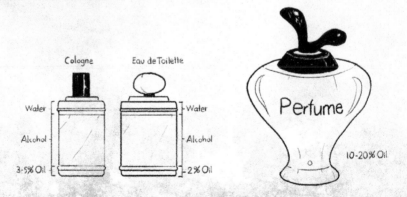

TYPES OF FRAGRANCES

note is the strongest but is the shortest lived. The middle note is more subtle and will last for several hours. The base or bottom note is the most subtle and will continue throughout the day. The base and middle note are what contribute to perfume's long life when compared with cologne. Cologne has only one layer (possibility two), and as such will not smell as strongly or last as long.

The misnomer of perfume being for women and cologne being from men likely arises from the scents that are typical of each product. A select perfume will usually consist of select flowery fragrances such as lavender, sandalwood, and eucalyptus. Colognes typically have a muskier odor, likely due to a contribution by a mammal called the civet cat, which lends a compound called civet. Castoreum, from beavers, and the musk of a male musk deer are also often used. Products utilized in both colognes and perfumes include the well known ambergris, a waxy substance derived from sperm whales.

Perfumes, unlike colognes, consist of several types: perfume, eau de parfum, eau de toilette, eau de cologne, and eau de fraiche. While each of these possesses different qualities, the most striking difference is their different concentrations of essential oils in comparison to the rest of their contents. Cologne consists of a weak scent and does not have to be diluted in such a manner. Colognes do have several subcategories as well, such as perfume pour homme, cologne, aftershave, and splash. As is evident by the names, most of these products simply have different uses rather than a different potency such as the perfumes. Due to the concentration of essential oils in colognes versus perfumes, it is usually assumed that a perfume will remain on the body for six to eight hours while a cologne is much more short-lived and only remains on the body for up to two hours. These concentrations of essential oils are also what make up the price difference between the two.

TYPES OF PERFUME CHART

Use the following chart as a quick reference guide for determining the proper ratio of essential oil, alcohol, and water when creating your fragrant product.

Fragrance Type	% oil	% alcohol	distill water or distillate
Extrait de Parfum/Perfume	15-40 (20% typical)	60-85	0-10
Esprit de Parfum	15-30	70-85	0-10
Eau de Perfume	10-15 (15% typical)	75-90	10-20
Eau de Toilette	5-15 (10% typical)	65-85	10-20
Eau de Cologne	3-5 (5% typical)	70	25-30
Eau de Fraiche	1-3 (2% typical)	80	15-20
Room or Linen Spray	3-7	20-30	63-77
Aftershave	2-5	75-83	15-20

From light as air to full on fragrant, your fragrance can vary whether it's a body splash containing only 8% perfume, or be slightly stronger as an eau de cologne with 3-5% perfume. Eau de toilette and solid perfumes like a balm may contain up to 30-40% perfume. And, depending on your personal preference, your own eau de parfum may deliver 15-30% perfume, while straight parfum is the strongest with up to 40% perfume.

FRAGRANCE COMPOSITION OF NOTES

Perfume or Parfum Extrait	Eau de Parfum	Eau de Toilette
Top Note: 20%	Top Note: 40%	Top Note: 50%
Middle Note: 30%	Middle Note: 30%	Middle Note: 30%
Base Note: 50%	Base Note: 30%	Base Note: 20%

Eau de Cologne	Eau de Fraiche
Top Note: 90%	Top Note: 70%
Middle Note: 10%	Middle Note: 20%
Base Note: 0%	Base Note: 10%

NUMBER OF DROPS EXAMPLE

Let's say you wanted to make a Parfum using a 10ml atomizer bottle. First determine how many drops your bottle holds, which in this case is 200 drops (20 drops per ml, so 20x10=200). For your perfume formula, you will be adding: 20% essential oil, 70% alcohol, and 10% distilled water. Since your essential oils comprise of 20% of the 200 drops, you will need 40 drops total of essential oil. The alcohol is 70% of the total 200 drops, which comes to 140 drops. The distilled water is 10% of 200 drops or 20 drops. These added together give you the total: 40 (oils) + 140 (alcohol) + 20 (water) = 200 drops.

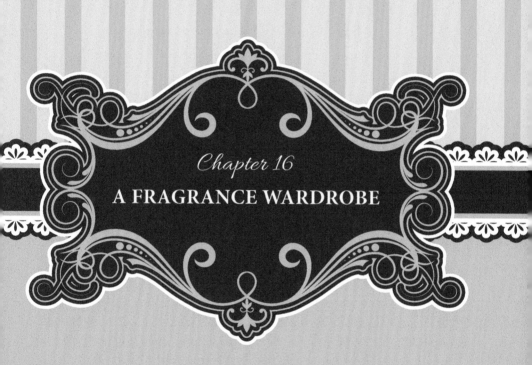

Chapter 16

A FRAGRANCE WARDROBE

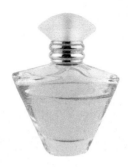

Perfume puts the finishing touch to elegance—a detail that subtly underscores the look, an invisible extra that completes a woman's personality. Without it there is something missing.

– GIANNI VERSACE

Perfumers understand just how emotionally evocative fragrances can be—from boosting your mood, to influencing those around you. Catching the whiff of a familiar aroma can trigger memories of particular people, places or experiences in the past. Naturally, these memories may have either positive or negative connotations, so it is important to discover a perfume that appeals to your own individual aromatic preferences.

Every time you wear a perfume, it will influence your mood, so it is worth taking the time to find one that you truly love. There is little point in wearing a perfume endorsed by your favorite celebrity, for example, if you do not find the aroma particularly pleasing. Perceptions of smell vary widely between people, so do not force yourself into liking a perfume just because it is popular, or on sale at half price. To one person, the scent of lavender may be comforting and remind them of their dearly-loved grandmother; to another, it may bring back painful memories of a strict, merciless teacher from their school days.

HOW DO I PICK THE RIGHT PERFUME?

One of the biggest mistakes a person makes when choosing a perfume is picking one without regard for the season or time of day. As a guideline, always select light and fresh perfumes for warmer months, because the hot weather can cause a fragrance heavy in florals to be overpowering. Wearing light, airy fragrances will prevent this. That being said, in the winter, you can wear heavier scents as these tend to last longer and don't come across as too strong. During the day, it is best to wear floral scents because they are much more accommodating in workplaces. In the evening, you can opt for a deeper scent such as orientals.

For those times you know you are going to be moving around a lot—in sports, for example—it might be best to have a sports fragrance. These fragrances are made to handle your sweat, complementing it, rather than becoming overpowering by it. Having a fragrance that is a bit spicy or citrus-like will help invigorate your senses and give you an energy rush every time you smell it.

One of the most common times to wear a fragrance is when you go out for the evening, for a night on the town. This is when you really need to give your fragrance wardrobe some thought. Several fragrances are perfect for the evening. Scents with a bit of musk or vanilla in them are pleasing to the senses and can be sensual. You also want a fragrance for the night that will stick around, not evaporate in an hour. Choose one that is long-lasting, so you stay smelling good for hours to come.

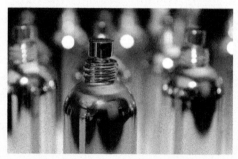 Selecting a fragrance wardrobe is all about you. Choose the right one for yourself in each situation, so that you can be sure your scent goes well with your wardrobe, and that you are not left standing alone because your fragrance is overpowering the room.

A fragrance is like a dress, an expression of personality.
It can be both erotic or powerful, or both, but it always
combines femininity and sensuality.
– Gianfranco Ferre, designer

You will be able to experiment with a combination of aromatic groups to create an overall effect, whether it is exotic and rich, or fresh and clean.

Creating a fragrance wardrobe may be a new idea to some. Think of it as how you have different clothes to suit an occasion; there are those who want to have a scent that suits occasions as well. This is what a fragrance wardrobe is all about.

Now that we know what it is, how do you go about creating it? There are several steps to doing so.

First, your fragrance should be dictated by the season you are wearing it in. For example, in hot weather, the fragrance will be impacted in two ways. The first way is that the heat causes you to sweat, which causes the scent to disappear off your skin as your sweat evaporates it into the air. Hot weather can take a fragrance away very quickly. The second issue is that hot weather will cause your fragrance to become stronger. The heavier of a fragrance you wear, the more likely it is to become overpowering. In the winter, choose to have a heavier fragrance because the opposite, of course, can be true for winter. Take these notes into consideration when choosing your fragrances for summer and winter.

WHAT IS YOUR PERFUME PERSONALITY?

Guerlain was reported to have said in 2005 that "perfumes are thought to have personalities," and with this in mind, let's explore the groups of perfumes different characters may gravitate towards.

Two leading authorities can contribute this, and offer a unique dimension. In 1949, American perfumer R. W. Moncrieff published his study, "What is odor: a new theory," where he investigated how the molecule of a particular smell could have an impact on the olfactory system. He discussed how he felt introverted people had a keener sense of smell and so may choose lighter, fresher fragrances than those who are more extroverted. Moreover, those with louder and prouder personalities may gravitate towards the brighter colors of the spectrum including warm reds, ochres, and purples; quieter people opted for pinks and pale blues.

In their 1988 paper, "Is selection of perfume a matter of chance?" fragrance psychologists Mensing and Beck added depth to this thought suggesting that leanings such as favorite colors may have a very direct correlation with the kind of perfume a person may choose.

With that in mind, what sort of personality do you have?

FUN AND SPORTY

The sporty girl is laid back and low key. She has a quirky sense of humor and a quick smile. Her lean athletic frame is her most attractive attribute, which matches well with the fact she has little or no interest in makeup. Her healthy glow is all she needs to attract admiring glances.

Unlikely to want to stand out in a crowd, she wants her fragrance to complement her personality rather than shout for attention.

Her perfume is designed as a finale rather than the whole show. Green notes work beautifully for this lady as do oceanic and fruity blends.

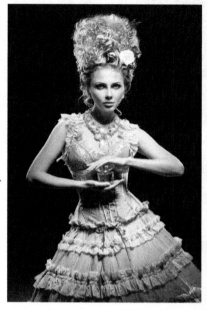

Women should have a wardrobe of scents that they change. It's not about putting on a pretty smell that you really like. You need to think specifically about what you want and how you want to feel—just as you do with your clothes. The French and Italians do that, yet I think we are quite scared about it. It's so much part of our outfit.

– Lyn Harris

OUTDOORS GODDESS

This girl thoroughly enjoys the richness of life. She loves nothing more than getting out in the countryside and feeling the wind stroke her hair.

She is warm and compassionate, has amazing empathy and is a wonderful friend.

This girl usually loves pale greens and light blues. Almost androgynous with her lean physique and physical strength, she may tend to gravitate not only to a quiet, unisex look in her clothes but in her fragrance choices, too.

She will have no truck with messing about creating a look because she has her very own air. She will want to complement rather than invoke a different personality. Eau de toilette or cologne will be her favorites, a simple spritz like fresh air. Oceanic, fruity and green blends are excellent for this lady. For a more sultry evening wear, woody chypre blends bring out the mystery and sensuality of this girl.

DYNAMIC AND IN CONTROL

You know her. She is bold; she has her finger on the pulse. When she walks into a room, people take notice. She has a spicy, fiery hot character. It is likely she loves the color purple especially since it is so closely aligned with royalty... because man, she loves the good life.

She loves dressing up, flirting and performing to a crowd. She is enigmatic having that "je ne sais pas." She can be a bit of a Machiavellian creature, liking to stir things up a bit and to break some rules.

This girl is excited by the dissonant harmonies of jazz and will always seek out exotic and enigmatic holidays.

For this girl, impact is the watchword. Her perfume choices will be about invoking a character, playing a part. Whether that is the dominatrix in the board room or the femme fatale, she will have a different scent for each. She loves exotic oriental blends and the headier the effect, the better. Wearing rich eau de parfum, there is no missing the sexuality or power of this vixen.

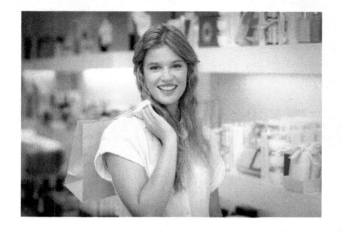

*A woman
should wear
perfume
wherever she
wants to be
kissed.*
— Coco Chanel

THE GIRLY GIRL

For the most feminine lady, floral fragrances are queen. They bring out the romantic nature of this girl who tends to be flirty and playful. Very sweet and vivacious, you will have guessed she loves pink and loves nothing more to be surrounded by flowers and beautiful things.

She will most often gravitate to woody florals, which are perfect for concerts listening to her favorite classical music. Simple, single notes are bewitching, especially when layered through her long, luxurious hair.

The girly girl's scent needs to be light and airy, playful like a dance on the air. To achieve this, go for a lighter eau de cologne and layer with body lotions and hair perfumes.

THE GIRL NEXT DOOR

Certainly, she's no plain Jane—this is the girl a boy happily takes home to his mom! Perhaps a little shy, she has an understated sexiness, which is utterly irresistible.

Perhaps even a little bit of a tom boy, research suggests she may have a penchant for the color yellow and you will likely hear her car radio belting out a bit of R&B. This girl loves a bit of luxury, but it is for her rather than the effect it will create.

Fruity scents work well for daytime wear; perhaps a light eau de toilette? In the evening, though, she likes to turn on the glamour and the contrast in her personality is often striking. Floral chypres bring out her femininity and create a sense of mystery, which she revels in.

There are many ways to wear perfume, and different ways to apply it depending on the type of perfume, as well as different scents that are appropriate for various settings. Perfume application, while seemingly simple, can become incredibly complex when one realizes that the manner and strength of application are supposed to differ based on weather, hormones, and stress. In addition to that, how someone prepares their skin can have a profound effect on the potency and effect of the perfume. Perfume also combines with the chemicals in a person's skin, and, as such, will smell different on different people. To select a perfume, it should be

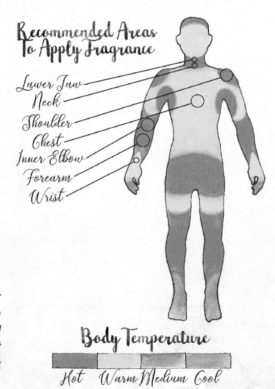

Recommended Areas To Apply Fragrance

Lower Jaw
Neck
Shoulder
Chest
Inner Elbow
Forearm
Wrist

Body Temperature

Hot Warm Medium Cool

When applying your perfume, do so before dressing. This will avoid leaving any permanent stains on fabric, pearls or metals.

sprayed on the skin and allowed to sit for ten to fifteen minutes so it can adequately mix with your body chemistry.

Perfume is best applied to clean, mostly dry skin. It is advisable to come from a warm shower so the pores are open and the perfume can be adequately soaked up by the skin, similar to how using a facial cleanser and shaving are best done in a warm shower since the warm water and humidity opens up the pores. When showering, it's advantageous to select a non-deodorizing soap and shampoo, as perfume has a tendency to mix with other scented products and this can dilute or completely change the smell of the perfume. For the same reason, spraying perfume over an area that has had lotion spread over it is not advised. Some suggest using a fragrance-free moisturizer to make the fragrance last longer on the skin. Or, you may want to apply unscented aloe vera gel before applying the perfume. This will help the fragrance molecules cling to your skin longer and keep you from having to reapply your scent later in the day.

When actually applying the perfume, it is usually sprayed in regions called "pulse points." These pulse points include the wrists, back of the knees, throat, behind the elbow, and behind your ears. These points are areas where blood flow is 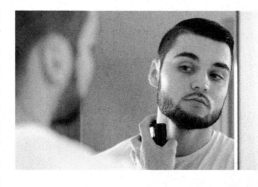 the strongest and skin is the warmest. Warm skin helps to emanate the perfume through the air, helping the scent create an aura around you, so someone doesn't have to come up and sniff your wrist to enjoy the smell of your perfume.

Avoid rubbing your wrists together after application, as this will crush the chemical and change the scent. Some people like to apply their perfume to their hair, and this is best done not by actually spraying the hair, but by spraying the brush. After spraying the brush with perfume, lightly brush through your hair a few times, and it will be appropriately scented. Some people choose to apply perfume by spraying it into the air and walking back and forth through the mist. When people select this method, a lot of product is wasted, but they feel they get a better all-over scent. In this case, only spray the perfume one or two times at most. Otherwise, the scent will be too strong and repel people rather than attract them.

When wearing perfume, it is important to consider the environment you'll be wearing it in and how the scent will affect others. If dressing for work in a small office, try not to select a strong perfume as it will overpower your coworkers. When traveling by public transportation, apply your perfume when you've arrived at your destination. Keep in mind, less is best. You want your scent to be amazing in an understated way, not like you bathed in it.

THE BEST WAY TO APPLY PERFUME

Although it may seem like common sense, there are some tips to applying perfume. It can be a very expensive purchase, so applying it right can save you money and product.

1. Targeted sprays of perfume are more efficient than walking through a spray of mist.
2. Applying a dab to the back of the knees will leave the scent behind you throughout the day.
3. Applying a dab to the chest will allow you to smell it throughout the day.
4. A bit to the wrist lets you take your scent whenever you want throughout the day.
5. After applying the perfume, let it dry rather than dabbing; this is recommended to keep the scent more intact.
6. When using a perfume that your pour out, you do not want to place the bottle against the skin and turn it upside down. This can allow for skin and oil particles to enter the bottle. Instead, moisten the stopper with the perfume and apply it to the skin. Then, clean the stopper and replace it.

Enigmatic fragrance results can be concocted using techniques that perfumers call layering. It is a practice about which the scent world is divided. Experimentalists reel at the prospect of the myriad of new experiences to savor. However, purists in their field remain unconvinced.

Feeling that the months of labor taken to create the finality of a scent should be revered, they shake their heads at their perceived desecration of their art. Still, though, it garners more and more followers and layering has become something of a trend.

The perfume wearer is able to obtain an entirely unique effect by wearing two different scents together. The stronger of the two fragrances is applied first, allowing the scent to dry down and letting the heart and base notes of the two perfumes to blend. Likewise, it is possible to layer textures, such as using a body lotion in one scent and layering over a second lighter one, too.

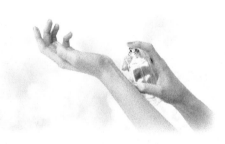

The art of the blending is in the selections of the fragrances. A citrus scent is by far the most adaptable. Use it to mingle with floral notes to make a pretty garden scent or with woody ones for a summer woodland scent. The richness of amber scents also makes a beautiful mix with citrus head notes. Full-bodied, these blends are robust and yet complement each other and are able to avoid being overpowering.

The layering, of course, causes overlaps in the floral makeup, enhancing the aroma of the head note even more. Think about the initial aroma. Tresor by Lancôme, in essence, is a rose and peach-scented perfume. Because the violet and amber oils have been blended in, it lost its overly sweet cosmetic edge, and the addition of jasmine and musk give it a modern twist on the summer garden scent. Add Crabtree and Evelyn Rose to it, though, and the balance will shift, bringing in a more virginal and innocent aura to it.

Adding a violet note brings a more mystical edge. Blended with Violette (Berdoues or Floris), it takes on a more ethereal and elusive feel and becomes tantalizing and yet unobtainable. The base note is heavier, and somehow it takes on a melancholy key. The sandalwood seems to become far defined as does the musk as the layers in both perfumes meld.

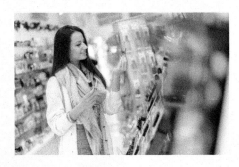

Green notes, in particular, make gorgeous combinations with oriental vanilla notes. The leathery depth of Yves Rocher Vanille Noire blends beautifully with the green notes of Dior Granville. The strong pine notes seem to neutralize the sweetness of the vanilla and bring out the orange blossom heart note. This fresh and dulcet fragrance is beautiful by day, contrasted with the spiciness of a nighttime blend of Vanille Noire and Guerlain's Shalimar. The spiciness of the cedarwood, orange blossom, and vanilla blended with the iris, jasmine, and rose of Guerlain's masterpiece invokes an exotic scent from souks wafting across desert sands.

Heady scents can take on a whole new dimension if you add to them a light citrus edge. Amarige de Givenchy is a traditional rich and heavy fragrance, but add Citrus Verbena by L'Occitane, and it entirely loses its cloying edge. While the heady heart notes of the tuberose and ylang ylang are still very much in the air, the cedarwood of the two products comes to the fore and the sharpness of the grapefruit and verbena balances it out.

It's a fascinating foray in previously uncharted waters in perfumery. Not only is it an opportunity to experiment and melt together two different scent worlds, it is also a chance to resurrect fragrances you may have long forgotten.

Old bottles of scent left dusty and unused suddenly have a whole new opportunity to sparkle again. They can add structure and substance to your designs. Those scents which previously you may have avoided as a little sickly sweet may now have a brand new purpose for you to discover. Layering holds the key.

SKIN CHEMISTRY

Have you ever noticed that your favorite perfume smells different on you than on your friend? Or, while you are taking medication, all of your perfumes smell differently on you now?

Some may claim that skin chemistry has nothing to do with the way your perfume smells on you, while others claim it has everything to do with the way it smells on you. Either way, all that really matters is how it smells on the skin. Some perfumers want to smell it on as many subjects as possible before determining its final composition.

It is really no surprise, since the skin has a chemistry and scent all its own. Factors that may contribute to these differences in scent could be a person's diet, lifestyle, medication, alcohol consumption and overall health. Another factor is one's skin type. For instance, dry skin may not absorb the citrus notes as quickly as another skin type.

You will want to try your fragrance out on several different people and note the differences in the way your perfume develops on their skin. The top note is where you may see the most noticeable change as well as throughout the drydown.

WHY DOES A FRAGRANCE SMELL GOOD ON MY FRIEND AND NOT ON ME?

Every person has a unique chemical makeup within their skin. This combination is composed of fats, proteins, water, fatty acids, salts, sugars, and fiber. The

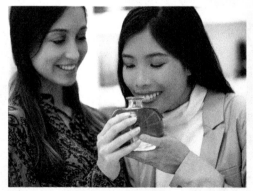

makeup of the skin can be affected by humidity, diet, hormones, stress and medications. You can see that each person has a different makeup than other people, as well as themselves from day to day. The fragrance reacts differently when the skin has more water, oil, collagen or other variables.

Most perfumes are a blend of chemicals evaporating at different speeds, which are affected by the skin makeup. This can cause a variance in the way a fragrance smells; if a friend had put the perfume on hours before you did, for example, you might detect a dominance of different chemicals than when first applied. For these reasons, it is recommended you experiment with fragrances on your own skin and see how they smell after a few hours to find the best fit for your unique makeup.

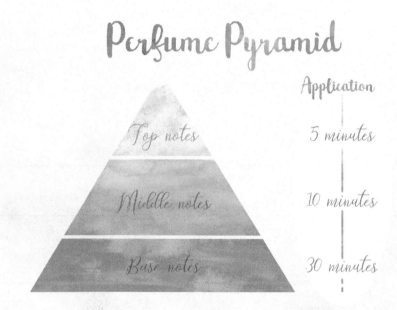

Perfume Pyramid

	Application
Top notes	5 minutes
Middle notes	10 minutes
Base notes	30 minutes

WHY DOES MY PERFUME WEAR OFF SO FAST?

The length a fragrance remains on the skin is dependent on the rate it evaporates. When the skin is dry, the fragrance will evaporate faster. If the skin has moisture in it, that will evaporate in combination with the perfume. This causes the scent to last longer in the cells. By applying a fragrance-free base of moisturizer to the skin, you can increase the amount of time it takes for the fragrance to evaporate. Applying the fragrance to hair and clothes can also help to hold the scent longer.

HOW DO I REMOVE PERFUME FROM MY SKIN?

If you were out for a fragrance testing and when you get home want to get a scent off, use these tips to remove it.

1. Use alcohol swabs to wipe the area.
2. Apply either a neutral base or unscented deodorant to the area, and then wash it off with laundry detergent.
3. Rinse with warm water.

Some perfumes are so strong that they tend to stick around for a couple of weeks. Fragrances to be careful with because of their long-lasting effects are musks.

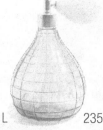

A FRAGRANCE WARDROBE

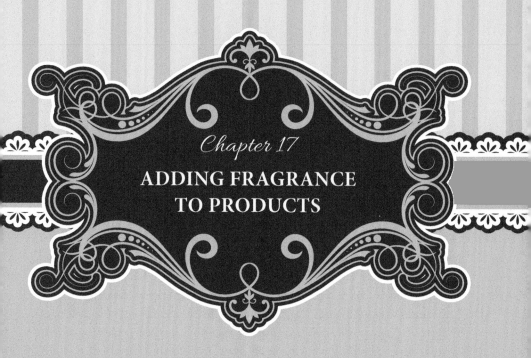

Chapter 17

ADDING FRAGRANCE
TO PRODUCTS

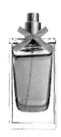

Perfume is the most intense form of memory.

– JEAN PAUL GUERLAIN

We all love the fragrance of our favorite shampoo or soap and more often that not choose that brand because of the way it smells. When creating your own product line, you may want to use the same fragrance for different products. However, a fragrance used in shampoo may not smell the same when used in a body lotion or cream. To avoid this, the percentages in the fragrance may be adjusted to cover the variations in base odor. Some reactions that may appear include a change in the look and consistency of your product. Too much adjustment of the fragrance formula may also cause varying reactions when applied to the skin.

Fragrances are primarily essential oil-based although some may be water-based and a non-ionic solubilizing surfactant such as polysorbate 20 or 80 may be used. The amount of solubilizer needed will vary from product to product; the general rule is to use three to four times the amount of solubilizer to fragrance and add fragrance to the surfactant before adding to the final product. Be sure to add your fragrance at the end of the formulation process. Adding your formula too early, while the product is still warm, could cause negative consequences. The more volatile components of the fragrance could evaporate off if still hot. This could also cause the fragrance not to smell as you expected. If heating is not required, the fragrance can be added during the oil phase of your formula.

It is important to test your product's stability, especially if you are planning on reselling your products to the public. Some fragrances may change the appearance of your product (especially clear gels) and cause them to look cloudy, hazy or even yellow. They can also cause the emulsion to separate or go grainy. Adding fragrance to a product may make it thinner, especially in shampoos and body washes. When this happens, you might want to add a pinch of salt to the final product after the fragrance has been added. Be sure to test your blend in a small amount of base before making larger amounts. This is a process of trial and error, and results will vary.

Since you will be working with natural fragrances that contain many reactive groups, carrying out a stability test will be necessary. Testing should be performed including storage under conditions of high heat. This will allow you to see how increased heat may drive potential reactions that may change the scent and color of a product. One possible solution to help with heat stability is to add an antioxidant to your products such as Vitamin E. The antioxidants in Vitamin E can react with the free radicals to neutralize their ability to react.

Intense lighting is another factor to consider and should be tested. Some fragrances are sensitive to light and exposure to light may turn a formula yellow or make it smell foul. When packaging, the type of plastic the product is eventually stored in should be carefully selected as it can also change the odor of the product. PET plastic is one type of plastic that can be used with fragrance. In cases where the fragrance is sensitive to light, a dark-colored container should be used.

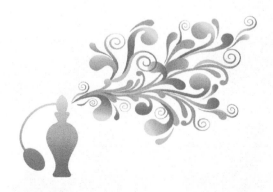

TIPS FOR PRESERVING PERFUMES
& NATURAL BODY CARE PRODUCTS

When you make your own organic products that are natural GMO-free alternatives for skin, body, and healthcare, you may be plagued with not knowing the shelf-life of your homemade creations. Creating safe alternatives to store-bought products can sometimes prove quite difficult.

Most people are not strangers to allergies like drying, irritation or in worst case scenarios, a skin disease caused by using conventional shampoos, soap, pastes, and cleaners and as a result, more people are opting for natural products that pose less threat to health. However, although the thought of buttering our bodies up with these items are worrisome especially with the potential health risks, can we really live without these preservatives? Well…let's find out how.

Where there is water, you will always find life, even in its basic form. Hence, it is a general rule that water-based creations will have a much shorter shelf-life than oil and butter-based creations. This is the magic behind the longevity and stability of salves and balms versus lotions and creams. Water-based products like insect repellents, linen sprays, and hair rinses are better produced in small batches as it not only helps prevent spoilage but also ensures the freshest ingredients are in use whenever you need them.

Although the natural ways to help add stability to home crafted skin and body care products may not be as long-lasting or equivalent to chemical commercial preservatives, the good news is you can create small batches to use up quickly or choose some natural preservatives to include in your creations. The key lies in understanding your ingredients and process.

1. KEEP YOUR CONTAINERS CLEAN

Sterilization is key here; most people assume powerful preservatives are all they need when in reality simple measures like ensuring all storage jars are clean can make a world of difference. A dishwasher does an excellent job of sterilizing and cleaning containers. Recycled containers for example should be washed with soap and water, a douse of vinegar and complete drying before usage ensures that your containers are no breeding ground for bacteria. Ensure there are no bits of food or other particles in containers before you use them. This also applies to oil infusions as bacteria and moisture can make oils go rancid fast. Even if the containers are new, it is advisable you wash before use.

If you make a lot of salves, lotions, and balms, consider having designated equipment. For example, a special stainless steel pot that you can dedicate to just soap making, or a blender, wooden spoon, spatula, and Pyrex measuring bowl that can be committed to body care products. Ensure you keep product supplies tidy and together in a lidded storage container. Another preventive measure is clean hands. Give your hands/fingers a good wash before dipping them into the mixture. Putting dirty hands into jars of salve or lotion will introduce bacteria and shorten the shelf-life.

2. STORAGE

- Serums should be stored in a cobalt or amber bottle rather than clear jars or bottles. This is because the dark color helps reduce the effect of light which speeds up deterioration. In fact, it is advisable to keep creations away from direct light whether they are subject to temperature fluctuations or not.
- Solid perfumes should not be stored in warm or hot places as they are also subject to temperature fluctuations. These creations tend to melt in warm conditions.
- Infused oils and vinegars, as well as ingredients such as butter and beeswax, should be stored in cool, dry places. Straining plant material from your infusions before storing, will also help them to last longer.
- For a warm or humid climate, or the heat of summer, some creations—particularly water-based ones should be stored in the fridge if you intend to keep them around for a while. Storage during summer or in warm climates is a lot more difficult than during a long, cold winter.

3. USE ANTIOXIDANTS AS PRESERVATIVES

When exposure to air or oxygen starts to compromise the oils or other ingredients, the process is known as oxidation. Although antioxidants are not actual preservatives, they do help to slow the oxidation process in ingredients that are prone to oxidation. A good example of antioxidants is Vitamin E Oil and Rosemary Antioxidant oil, which serve as natural stabilizers. They can be included in homemade serums, perfume oils, solid perfume recipes, etc., to help elongate or extend shelf life. However, they best added to the oil base, or after the oil base has been mixed with melted waxes and butters. Avoid heating them directly.

4. USE ESSENTIAL OILS AND ALCOHOL AS PRESERVATIVES

Like antioxidants, essential oils, hydrosols, vegetable gycerine, tinctures and alcohol extracts can help inhibit the growth of bacteria and other unsavory micro-organisms. However, you may have to work on a formula especially when using alcohol as alcohol doesn't mix well with all fats, and also remember to only add your essential oils at the end of a preparation.

5. USE DISTILLED, BOILED WATER OR WATER-SUBSTITUTES

Distilled water helps purify your preparation process as it kills some bacteria that may be present in water. Tea or water infusions, aloe vera gel, witch hazel extract, hydrosols, and vegetable glycerine are all water-based, hence using distilled or boil water before including it in recipes can help eliminate possible contaminants. Refrigerating these items can also help to extend the shelf-life and keep both these ingredients and your creations fresher longer.

UNDERSTAND THE NATURE OF YOUR INGREDIENTS

Different oils and butter can be heated to high temperatures while others can be both a solid and a liquid. Understanding the shelf-life of your ingredients and how they react with other ingredients can help tailor down your recipes to suit body care or health needs. It also helps you anticipate the storage conditions. One of the main the reasons why people opt for natural and organic body care products is to avoid the array of synthetic chemicals found in commercial ones; therefore it is important to always remember that while you can add some preservatives to your creations, you cannot have the same shelf-life as those that are mass-produced. The best way to enjoy your natural creations is to craft in small batches and use them up while the ingredients are still fresh.

Chapter 18

PRETTY PACKAGING

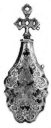

*Smell is a potent wizard that transports you
across thousands of miles and all the years
you have lived.*

– Helen Keller

In the fragrance industry, more than any other industry, the need for great packaging is key. The bottle you choose not only contains the elixir of the dream but extends everything you want to convey about the brand and the promise it makes.

There are practical considerations as well. A spray bottle or atomizer, for instance, will limit the amount of oxygen exposure the blend gets and so will enhance the shelf life. But when it comes to choosing which pretty bottle is best, how does one choose?

Clearly, fragrance houses spend exorbitant amounts of money perfecting this stage of production, but are bespoke bottles the only option? Given they are extremely expensive and add lengthy steps to your process, they add a hefty margin to your price tag. Often with a little imagination and savoir faire, it can be possible to customize off-the-shelf designs easily and effectively.

First, analyze who your target buyer is. The bottle designed for the hip teenager will be markedly different from that aimed at the luxury men's market, for instance. What is the feel of the scent; what is its message? Should it be romantic and opulent to the touch, or is it a no-frills, very light appeal? The bottle should echo the sentiment.

How does the shape of the bottle knit with the feel of your brand? Not only are there different sizes to choose from but square, rectangular and cylindrical bottles are easy to come by and of course come in a range of colors, too.

When it comes to customization of the bottle, it is possible to create individuality through a million different ways. What can be restrictive is a strangely shaped bottle. The simpler the basic shape of the glass the more freedom to be interesting you have. Opt for a bottle that has a lovely wide surface so you can really go to town with your artwork.

Labels are not your only friend; stoppers and caps come in a wide variety of designs. Choose a bottle with a neck of FEA 15 to be able to exploit this opportunity to its fullest. Why not consider adding a charm to add luxury or shells to echo an oceanic blend?

At all points remember that the whole point of perfume is that it is a sensory experience. Some of the most compelling trends for packaging are where the texture is also involved. You may want to use a wooden box or a velvet bag—the possibilities are endless.

From a technical standpoint, you must also go for a bottle that gives you a margin of error outside of your labeled capacity. In the heat, alcohol expands, so ensure you leave space for this process to happen naturally and then return to its normal size.

WHAT IS A DECANTER BOTTLE?

Decant, as defined by Webster's dictionary, is to pour from one vessel into another. As a perfumer, you will be transferring your product by pouring or using sterile pipettes to take perfume from its original large decanter bottle and repackage it in a smaller bottle for a customer.

SHELF LIFE FOR NATURAL PERFUMES

Ideally, perfumes should last approximately two to three years. Even after this time, it technically doesn't go "bad," but the top notes tend to dissipate leaving it with less sillage than when first created. Storing your perfume properly is the best way to prolong the life of your perfume. Industry professionals recommend replacing your perfume every year.

CHOOSING THE RIGHT PERFUME BOTTLE

Choosing the right bottle for your perfume is imperative, regardless if it is just for personal use or for retail. You will want to use dark glass bottles for storing your perfumes, floral waters, and colognes. Old perfume bottles purchased at garage sales or flea markets can be utilized as well, if thoroughly washed with hot, soapy water, and rinsed with isopropyl alcohol and dried before filling. Be sure to inspect old bottles carefully to make sure no residue lingers in the bottom of the bottle and that the top fits properly. If the bottle has a screw top, be sure the liner inside the cap is there so contents do not come into contact with the plastic or leak out.

For lesser-concentrated splashes, you can use plastic bottles with snug-fitting caps. However, stronger concentrations require glass containers. Bottles made from HDPE will collapse if filled with perfume, perfume oil, eau de parfum, or cologne. Spray bottles work well for splashes, room/linen sprays, and floral waters or hydrosols.

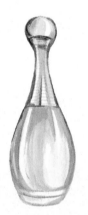

To purchase bottles in bulk, please check the resource section in the back of this book. You can find inexpensive bottles at beauty supply or dollar stores locally.

Type of Container	Type of Use
Glass	Perfumes, Perfume Oils, Eau de parfum, Cologne
PVC or PET (polyvinyl chloride or polyethylene terephthalate plastic)	Massage Oils, Bath Oils
HDPE (high-density polyethylene)	Body Lotions, Creams, Toners, Facial Sprays
Tins	Solid Perfumes, Salves

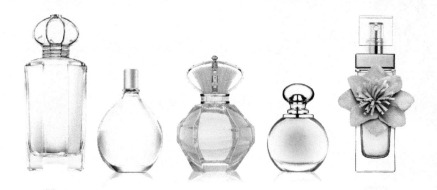

BRANDING YOUR SCENT

If you are considering starting a home business selling your product line, you will need to find a more uniform look for your containers. How you package your fragrance will help convey your brand and the idea or message behind your scent. The visual aspect of the package will be a key factor in persuading consumers to choose yours over another. This is where you do NOT want to cut corners. Spend time comparing packaging online see what resources are available in developing the bottle that can make your product stand out. Your marketing plan for your product line will need to take into consideration your brand values, target audience, and fragrance type.

Alessandro Prestini, CEO of Quadpack perfumery partner Premi says, "Brand is everything in the fragrance world. A perfume pack can take different shapes, colors, and finishes. The decoration possibilities are endless, but what matters is that the look and feel are right for the brand. A fragrance bottle for the teenage market will look vastly different from a bottle aimed at professional men."

Visit any major department store's beauty counter to get some ideas. What catches your eye? Is there anything that immediately jumps out at you and draws you in? Think about what you find most appealing. As you can see, there are hundreds of options. Every major perfume brand on earth is competing for a slice of this multi-billion dollar industry. Interesting packaging will lure the customer to take a closer look and possibly take a whiff. But scent won't be the other factor when closing the sale; how the perfume looks in the bottle is the other part.

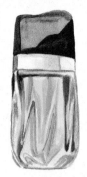

Think about this. You are at a craft fair, and there are two tables selling perfume. One table has some great-smelling perfumes, but they are all in glass containers used for canning vegetables. The other table has okay-smelling perfumes, but they are in beautiful glass bottles designed to look elegant. Which do you think will get more sales?

They say that you should never judge a book by its cover, but we do, and perfume sales reflect that. That is why it is so important that you choose the right perfume bottle. There are simple shapes on the market such as cylindrical, square, rectangular in various capacities such as 30, 50, 100-milliliter sizes. A standard bottle can be striking with a professional label with little investment. Experts suggest avoiding very strange shapes, and offering a more personalized, decorated bottle for a smarter, cleaner way to demonstrate your brand's personality. One of the key features to keep in mind is the bottle capacity. Alcohol can expand at high temperatures, so you will need to leave a margin.

Remember these tips when choosing a perfume bottle for your fragrance.

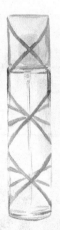

- First, look at the image you're projecting with your perfume, who your target audience is, and what type of fragrance you want to sell. This will dictate to you the shape, capacity and even the color of the bottle.
- While it can be fun to be unique, you should avoid having bottles that are in strange shapes. It is better to decorate and personalize a bottle, which presents your brand's personality in a smart way.
- One great tip is to make sure your bottleneck size is standard. That allows you a wider selection of caps that can really add to the personality of the bottle and your brand.

- Avoid tall, thin bottles. Choose large, flat containers that give you a greater area for decoration.
- Look at the different colors of glass for your perfume bottle. Choose one that doesn't make the perfume look bland in the bottle, but which also uses your company's own colors as well.
- Try adding a charm or ribbon for flair. This will give your product a look and feel of luxury. Garnishing your fragrance with a soft-touch finish adds to the emotional experience of the purchase.

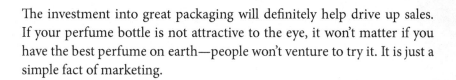

The investment into great packaging will definitely help drive up sales. If your perfume bottle is not attractive to the eye, it won't matter if you have the best perfume on earth—people won't venture to try it. It is just a simple fact of marketing.

WHAT IS THE BEST WAY TO STORE MY PERFUME?

Heat and light can reduce the life of perfume, so storing the bottle in a dark, cool place is best. Also, limit the amount of exposure the perfume has to air.

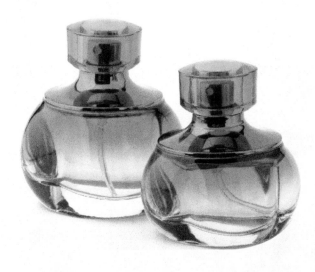

PRETTY PACKAGING

Chapter 19

FRAGRANCE REGULATIONS

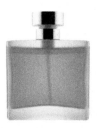

A woman's perfume tells more about her than her handwriting.

– Christian Dior

The fragrance industry is self-regulating, but it takes direction from the International Fragrance Association. While not a legislating body in their own right, their standards form the basis of the IFRA Code of Practice, which is deemed to be the globally recognized benchmark of ethics. Established in 1973, the IFRA has members from 100 manufacturing companies from 15 different countries.

One of the main parts of their job is to perform risk managements on each of the components that are used in perfumery. Some of these constituents may be entirely prohibited, others restricted.

The expert panel is made up not only of perfumers but also dermatologists, toxicologists and environmental consultants. As a group, they make recommendations on the safety of oils, particularly for skin sensitivity but also on the sustainability of plant and animal resources, which may be used in manufacture. Their website gives clear guidelines on which components to avoid and what potency is allowed on controlled substances.

The investigation into the safety of fragrance components is the responsibility of the Research Institute for Fragrance Materials (RIFM), who gather together their findings and then submit them to IFRA.

Testing only raw fragrance materials, since their inception in 1966 they have evaluated over 1,300 components. Their role is to check for any indications a component may be: sensitizing, neurotoxic, carcinogenic, phototoxic, photosensitizing, or may have biological effects. They may also advocate restriction measures should they feel they have insufficient information to make a judgment.

The Cosmetic Toiletry and Fragrance Association (CTFA) also have input in safety guidelines. Formed in 1894 with a massive 500 members, they are the loudest voice in the US personal care industry. Their role is to "protect the freedom to compete in a fair and responsible marketplace." As such, a third of their annual budget is spent in science relating to the industry and for lobbying government.

In 1976, the CTFA launched the Cosmetics Ingredients Review Board or CIR—a separate governing body, whose sole function is safety.

Interestingly, unlike other industries the regulation to some degree relies on the trust of the members, which presents its own challenges. There have been some examples of the shortfalls of this system. In 1977, it was found that AETT was neurotoxic to rats. Subsequently, it was found that a monograph had previously highlighted this when published by *Food and Chemical Toxicology*, but the findings had not been pinpointed. Consequently, AETT was discreetly withdrawn after having been used as an ingredient in many perfumes for over twenty years.

Musk Ambrette, too, has been assigned the status of being both phototoxic and neurotoxic, again after being earmarked by *Food and Chemical Toxicology*. In fact, even after the recommendations for withdrawal were made, a good five years elapsed before its removal was seen.

Further problems can come from trust issues further down the judicial ladder. Since the responsibility for the safety of products as outlined by the US Federal Drug and Cosmetics Act falls squarely at the manufacturers' feet, there are no checks made to safeguard the consumer outside of these guidelines.

Labeling, for instance, dictates the need for fragrances to be listed as ingredients. Since a formula, however, is seen to be a trade secret, it is not necessary to list all of the ingredients included. Therefore, should a perfumer want to take the risk of including some banned substance, it may be hard to control that action.

Many countries also have their own legislation pertaining to labeling, especially when it comes to cosmetics. In Europe, for instance, labeling falls under the judiciary of EU Regulation (EC) No. 1223/2009 and then is enforced by each country's own Trading Standards agency.

In short, then, the guidelines are not only vague but are also subjective to which country you decide to manufacture in.

HEALTH AND SAFETY AUDIT

As with any workplace, there are certain health and safety guidelines designed to ensure safe working environments. Most pertinent is COSHH, which is a British organization and overseas control of hazardous substances. Their procedures, when followed, give excellent insights into safe storage and handling of any components used in your process.

The two largest concerns in perfumery are always going to be skin reactions to oils used and the highly flammable alcohol base. Ventilation measures can make the difference between a day when the world goes swimmingly and an overwhelming headache. It makes good sense to undertake regular risk assessments. Your personal peace of mind is rested, but more importantly, having a folder of these can favorably impact insurance policies, too.

There is lots of appeal for corporate buyers of your products to have the reassurance of written guidelines about your processes and procedures. They want to see that the first product they buy from you can be replicated over and over, and their supply chain can be kept secure. Health and safety risk assessments form one of the most carefully thought-out aspects of your business and never fail to give a good impression.

ESSENTIAL OILS STORAGE AND SAFETY

Because essential oils contain no fatty acids, they are not susceptible to rancidity like vegetable oils, but you will want to protect them from the degenerative effects of heat, light, and air. Store them in tightly sealed, dark glass bottles away from any heat source. Properly stored oils can maintain their quality for years. (Citrus oils are less stable and should not be stored longer than six months after opening.)

ESSENTIAL OIL STORAGE TIPS

- Keep oils tightly closed and out of reach of children.
- Always read and follow all label warnings and cautions.
- Do not purchase essential oils with rubber glass dropper tops. Essential oils are highly concentrated and will turn the rubber to gum, thus ruining the oil.
- Make a note of when the bottle of essential oil was opened and its shelf life.
- Many essential oils will remove the furniture's finish. Use care when handling open bottles.
- Keep essential oil vials and clear glass bottles in a box or another dark place for storing.
- Be selective of where you purchase your essential oils. The quality of essential oil varies widely from company to company. Additionally, some companies may falsely claim their oils are undiluted and pure when they are not.

ESSENTIAL OIL SAFETY

In general, essential oils are safe to use for creating fragrances. Nonetheless, safety must be exercised due to their potency and high concentration. Please read and follow these guidelines to obtain the maximum effectiveness and benefits.

- To avoid getting essential oils in the eyes, wear protective eyewear. If you do happen to splash a drop or two of essential oil in the eyes, use a small amount of olive oil (or another carrier oil) to dilute the essential oil and absorb with a washcloth. For serious conditions, seek medical attention immediately.

- Store your essential oils and other raw materials out of reach from children.
- If a dangerous quantity of essential oil has been ingested, immediately drink olive oil and induce vomiting. The olive oil will help in slowing down its absorption and dilute the essential oil. Do not drink water—this will speed up the absorption of the essential oil.
- Never use oils undiluted on your skin. Pay attention to safety guidelines regarding certain essential oils, such as cinnamon and clove bud. These may cause skin irritation for those with sensitive skin. If you experience slight redness or itchiness, place olive oil (or any carrier oil) on the affected area and cover with a soft cloth. The olive oil acts as an absorbent fat and binds to the oil, diluting its strength and allowing it to be immediately removed. Aloe vera gel also works well as an alternative to olive oil. Never use water to dilute essential oil—this will cause it to spread and enlarge the affected area. Redness or irritation may last 20 minutes to an hour.
- For sensitive skin or when using a new oil, perform a "Skin Patch Test." If irritation occurs, discontinue use of such oil or blend. See section Skin Patch Test.
- If you are pregnant, lactating, suffer from epilepsy or high blood pressure, have cancer, liver damage, or another medical condition, use essential oils under the care and supervision of a medical practitioner.
- To prevent irritation to the skin while working with essential oils and absolutes, gloves and protective eyewear should be worn.
- Disposal of components should be handled properly in accordance with local regulations to avoid water pollution.
- When creating products, be sure to add a warning to the label, "Discontinue use if irritation occurs."

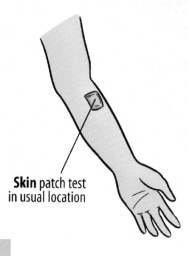

Skin patch test
in usual location

SKIN PATCH TEST

Certain essential oils can cause sensitization or an allergic reaction in some individuals. When using a new oil for the first time, you may want to perform a simple skin patch test on the inside of your arm or your chest. Place one drop of the essential oil into a carrier oil. Apply one drop on the skin and cover with a bandage. If skin becomes irritated and red, remove the bandage and immediately wash the area with soap and water. If after 12 hours no irritation has occurred, it is safe to use on the skin.

For someone who tends to be highly allergic, here is a simple test to determine if he or she is sensitive to a particular carrier oil and essential oil.

First, rub a drop of carrier oil onto the upper chest. In 12 hours, check for redness or other skin irritation.

If the skin remains clear, place 1 drop of selected essential oil in 15 drops of the same carrier oil, and again rub into the upper chest. If no skin reaction appears after 12 hours, it is safe to use the carriers and the essential oil.

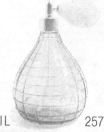

NATURAL PERFUME WITH ESSENTIAL OIL

UNDERSTANDING FRAGRANCE ALLERGIES AND COMMON SYMPTOMS

There are many types of fragrances categorized as either chemical or natural perfumes based on the ingredients used to make them. In most cases, the chemical scents are more toxic than their natural counterparts and may cause adverse allergies if not handled correctly. Below are some common allergic reactions that one may experience while using/handling these fragrances.

SYMPTOMS OF FRAGRANCE SENSITIVITY

Two types of allergic reactions caused by fragrance sensitivity include respiratory (runny eye and nose symptoms like that of a cold) and skin allergy symptoms. Other symptoms may include:

- Headaches
- Wheezing and/or difficulty breathing
- Tightness in the chest
- Stuffy or runny nose
- Sneezing
- Itchy skin, redness, or rash

Those with asthma or breathing difficulties may also find strong scents problematic due to the asthmatic symptoms they cause. The frequency of these allergic reactions has significantly increased over the last few years due to the production of more sophisticated perfumes, some of which contain exotic ingredients. A recent study performed by the University of West Georgia stated that over 30 percent of people surveyed said they found scented products irritating.

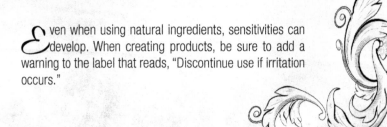

Even when using natural ingredients, sensitivities can develop. When creating products, be sure to add a warning to the label that reads, "Discontinue use if irritation occurs."

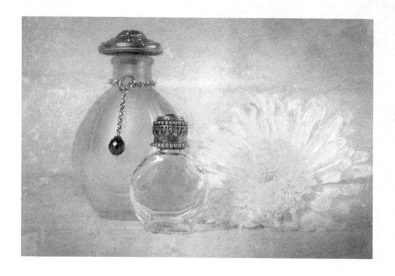

In medical terms, an allergy refers to a hypersensitive immune system where the body's defenses become hypersensitive and perceive any foreign substance, including fragrances, as a potential threat to the body. As such, the immune system is triggered to release a unique chemical known as histamine.

Histamine is often responsible for the perceptible reactions that you may see after being exposed to the fragrance, some of which include sneezing, headaches, nasal congestion, hives, skin rashes, peeling skin, and asthma, amongst others.

So, while some people may call it a "perfume allergy," it could be a fragrance sensitivity or an allergy to a particular chemical in a perfume.

CAUSES OF FRAGRANCE ALLERGY

Though many people blame specific fragrances for triggering allergic reactions, experts widely believe that these reactions are due to the harsh chemical composition of modern commercial scents. Therefore, an otherwise mild product that has been masked with lab-manufactured aromatic ingredients would trigger certain reactions.

However, researchers have not been able to forthrightly determine whether it's one compound or a combination of many compounds that is causing such allergic reactions. Some perfumes also have irritant effects and may cause choking and breathing difficulties, especially when there is excessive exposure to these compounds.

Among the wide selection of chemicals found in perfumes, only a few of them are suspected to trigger sensitivity or allergic reactions. Some of these chemicals are cinnamon alcohol, eugenol, cinnamon aldehyde, geraniol, oakmoss absolute and hydroxy citronellal.

Though these compounds are mainly used in making fragrances, they may also be found in household air fresheners. These chemicals may make you more susceptible to respiratory disorders. Furthermore, chemicals such as acetone, benzyl alcohol, camphor, ethyl acetate and ethanol can also cause irritation in your respiratory tract.

OTHER SYMPTOMS OF FRAGRANCE ALLERGY

The most common symptoms of sensitivity to a fragrance include sneezing, headaches, running nose, concentration problems, eczema, hives or skin rash. Mild nausea may also occur, which can make you vomit uncontrollably in case you have ingested food before being exposed to the fragrance. For most people, these symptoms usually disappear once the smell is out of their range, while for others the reactions are experienced more frequently and even become more intense with every repeated exposure.

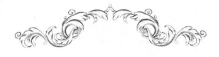

Though these allergies may appear somewhat similar to the symptoms of those caused by natural substances such as dander and pollen grains, experts are of the opinion that considerable differences exist between the two forms of allergy. In most natural ingredients, the immune system usually perceives allergens as

*I*t's advisable not to apply fragrances and perfumes when visiting public places such as your workplace as some people may show allergic reactions even if they may not appear to you. This would, in turn, affect their overall productivity rate. So, if people hold their noses when you're passing, know that the perfume you applied in the morning or have handled could be the problem.

invaders and releases antibodies to fight them back. However, some synthetic fragrance ingredients are so minimal and cannot be easily detected by one's body's defenses. Hence, when they reach the skin, they can totally modify it by binding up with the dermis. The body usually mistakes such modified proteins as foreign substances and may attack them indiscriminately, thus causing more severe allergic reactions.

Apart from the scented products, many fragrances-free substances may also trigger hypersensitivity since they contain imperceptible chemicals that one unknowingly inhales. Therefore, it's appropriate to do a patch test before handling a fragrance, thereby avoiding any major allergic symptoms. You can also visit a qualified dermatologist or physician to know more about any potential allergies, including any precautions that should be followed for preventing consecutive recurrences.

FRAGRANCE REGULATIONS

Chapter 20

BASIC RECIPES

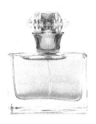

*A woman who doesn't wear perfume
has no future.*

– Coco Chanel

Now that you have a basic understanding of how to make perfume, follow these simple recipes as a guideline for preparing your own perfume products.

With these recipes, you can formulate a simple chord consisting of a top (head), middle (heart), and bottom (base) note or choose a different ratio proportion for a different effect. Some of the recipes below are based on blending by notes, but you can easily convert these recipes to use another method such as blending by aromatic family or accords.

Of course, there is plenty of room for creativity, as there are no hard and fast rules when it comes to creating your distinctive blend. You can add more or less. Feel free to change these to suit your own personal taste!

SOLID PERFUMES

While filling up your perfume containers with your favorite homemade perfume is fun and easy to do, you'll find that making solid perfume is even more satisfying. Most of the supplies for making solid perfume can be found at a craft and health food stores. Here is a checklist to take to the store, so you can get busy making your favorite scent solid perfume.

WHAT YOU WILL NEED:
    Small glass jar for mixing or Glass pyrex measuring cup
    Saucepan
    Glass stir rod
    Glass, stone, ceramic or a tin container for storing your perfume
    30 drops essential oils of your choice
    1/3 ounce Beeswax Beads
    1 Tablespoon Almond or Jojoba oil or Vitamin E

WHAT TO DO:
1. Add one tablespoon of Almond or Jojoba oil and 1/3 ounce of beeswax in the small glass jar.

2. Fill about 1-2 inches of water in a saucepan and place the glass jar with the oil and beeswax in it in the water. Bring the water in the saucepan to a boil to allow the wax to melt. When it's completed melted and liquid, remove it from the stove.

3. After the contents have cooled for about a minute, add approximately 30 drops of essential oils into the mixture. Stir with a glass stir rod, allowing as little as possible to stick to the rod, so not to waste any of your precious perfume. Make sure it's thoroughly mixed.

4. Pour your liquefied wax into your tin, glass or stone container and let it cool for at least 30 minutes. The mixture you've made

will make about one-half ounce of solid perfume, so you may need several tins or containers depending on their size.

5. If you find the solution too soft, you can remelt and add more beeswax beads.

6. To use your perfume once it has turned solid is simply rub your finger on the surface of the perfume and rub it on your neck, wrist or any place you desire.

You'll find that solid perfume is fun to make and you'll want to experiment with many different fragrances. These are great for great for traveling and can be put in a small container of your choice and carried in your purse or glove compartment. Be sure to try making several scents and share with friends as gifts.

EXOTIC FLORAL
15 drops Orange essential oil
7 drops Frankincense essential oil
8 drops Rose essential oil

CITRUS BLOSSOM
10 drops Lime essential oil
10 drops Neroli essential oil
10 drops Lemon essential oil

PUCKER UP
15 drops Lemon essential oil
10 drops Benzoin essential oil
5 drops Black Pepper essential oil

ORIENT EXPRESS
15 drops Bergamot essential oil
10 drops Ylang Ylang essential oil
5 drops Rose essential oil

BRIGHT AND EARLY
10 drops Lemon essential oil
15 drops Peppermint essential oil
5 drops Rosemary essential oil

FLORAL GARDEN
6 drops Lemon essential oil
7 drops Geranium essential oil
7 drops Lavender essential oil
10 drops Patchouli essential oil

PERFUME OILS

The ratio of essential oils to carrier oil can vary slightly when creating a natural perfume. As a general rule of thumb, you can use 80% carrier oil to 20% essential oils. Its always best to start with less and add more if you feel the scent is not strong enough. The old adage time will tell certainly is true in this case. When you allow your blend to mature, scents will meld together and change. This will be the time to determine whether more essential oils are necessary.

WHAT YOU WILL NEED:
  Glass Vial with Lid
  Glass Dropper
  Perfumer's Funnel
  120 drops Carrier oil (Fractionated Coconut, Almond, or Jojoba)
  30 drops Essential oils

WHAT TO DO:
1. Starting with a small glass vial, you can use a dropper to add your base note first, followed by the middle and top notes respectively.

2. Once you are satisified with the scent of your blend, you will want to add in your carrier oil. For this, you will need to add in four times the amount of the total essential oil blend. For instance, if you have a total of 30 drops of your top, middle, and base notes, you will need to add 120 drops of carrier oil to the final blend. Replace cap on vial.

3. Let blend sit for 24 hours in a dark, cool place. Check fragrance and adjust if necessary.

PERFUMES AND COLOGNES

The difference between perfumes and colognes will be the concentration and ratio of essential oils and alcohol. A cologne will be between 5-10% essential oil, while a perfume can be up to 20-30% essential oils. Getting your fragrance to have longevity (and last more than two hours on the skin) will be your one of your biggest challenges in perfume making. Here is where you will need to work out your own ratios based on the oils/accords chosen for your blend. Top head note range anywhere between 10-30% of your blend, Middle or heart notes make up 30-60% of your blend, and your base or bottom note can be 15-30% of your blend. Some perfumers use 30-50 different notes in a blend. Working with your accords and fixatives are key!

WHAT YOU WILL NEED:
    15 ml Dark glass bottle for storage
    Glass Dropper
    Funnel
    ½ ounce Perfumer's Alcohol
    30-90 drops Essential oils (30:40:30 ratio for top, middle, and base note is typical)

WHAT TO DO:
1. In a glass vial or bowl, add your essential oils starting with your base note followed by your middle note and top notes for your blend. You will want to build each accord separately before blending accords together.

2. Once you are satisfied with your accords, you can use a separate vial to combine your accords, one drop at a time.

3. If you find after adding your top notes that you need more of another note such as a base note, it is okay to go back and add more to balance it out.

4. After you finish your blend, you will want to test your blend on your skin, or use a perfume strip to smell it. Once satisfied, you will add your oils to the alcohol (percentage of alcohol used will depend on whether this is a perfume or cologne).

5. Using a funnel, add your perfume/cologne to a bottle and close with a cap. Let sit and macerate for a month or so in a dark, cool place. You can shake your blend 1-3 times a day.

6. If it is clear, you can bottle it right away. If your blend is hazy or cloudy after a checking it, you can filter it into a beaker (wet your filter with alcohol first before pouring your blend through), then bottle it.

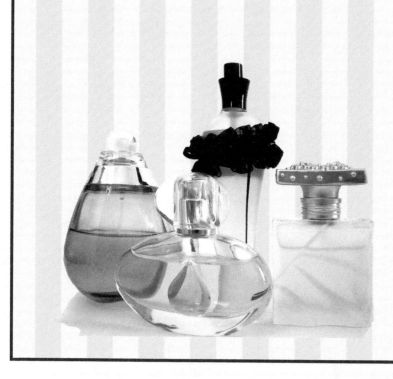

COLOGNES (WATER BASED)

In this recipe, distilled water is used along with alcohol for dilution. You can adjust the amount of water and alcohol used to increase or decrease its concentration.

WHAT YOU WILL NEED:
    30 ml Dark glass bottle for storage
    Glass Dropper
    Funnel
    4 ½ teaspoons Perfumer's Alcohol
    1 ½ teaspoon Distilled Water
    30 drops Essential oils

WHAT TO DO:
1. In a glass vial or bowl, add your essential oils starting with your base note followed by your middle note and top notes for your blend. You will want to build each accord separately before blending accords together.

2. Once you are satisfied with your accords, you can use a separate vial to combine your accords, one drop at a time, up to 30 drops of essential oil.

3. If you find after adding your top notes that you need more of another note such as a base note, it is okay to go back and add more to balance it out until you are satisfied.

4. After you finish your cologne blend, you will want to test your blend on your skin, or use a perfume strip to smell it. Once satisified, you will add your oils to the alcohol (percentage of alcohol used will depend on whether this is a perfume or cologne).

5. Using a funnel, add your perfume/cologne to a bottle and close with a cap. Let sit and macerate for a month or so in a dark, cool place.

6. Once you think your cologne is ready to bottle, check its clarity. If it is clear, you can bottle it right away. If your blend is hazy or cloudy, you will want to run your blend through a filter it into a beaker (wet your filter with alcohol first before pouring your blend through), then bottle it.

PERFUMES (WATER BASED)

In this recipe, distilled water is used along with alcohol for dilution. You can adjust the amount of liquid by increasing it, if you decide its too strong.

WHAT YOU WILL NEED:
  30 ml Dark glass bottle for storage
  Glass Dropper
  Funnel
  4 ½ teaspoons Perfumer's Alcohol
  1 ½ teaspoon Distilled Water
  60-90 drops Essential oils

WHAT TO DO:
1. In a glass vial or bowl, add your essential oils starting with your base note followed by your middle note and top notes for your blend/accord. You will want to build each accord separately before blending accords together.

2. Once you are satisfied with your accords, you can use a separate vial to combine your accords, one drop at a time, up to 90 drops of essential oil.

3. If you find after adding your top notes that you need more of another note such as a base note, it is okay to go back and add more to balance it out until you are satisfied.

4. After you finish your perfume blend, you will want to test your blend on your skin, or use a perfume strip to smell it. Once satisified, you will add your oils to the alcohol.

5. Using a funnel, add your perfume to a bottle and close tightly with a cap. Let sit and macerate for a month or so in a dark, cool place. You can shake your bottle up to three times a day to blend.

6. Once you think your perfume is ready, check its color. If it is clear, you can bottle it right away. If your blend is hazy or cloudy, you can pour your blend through a filter into a beaker (wet your filter with alcohol first before pouring your blend through), then bottle it.

BODY SPRAYS

The main difference between perfumes and body sprays is the amount of essential oils and water used. Body sprays are less concentrated with more liquid (hydrosol, water, or alcohol) and less essential oils. Body sprays have only four ingredients: alcohol, distilled water, essential oils, and glycerin. Witch hazel is not recommended since it only contains 14% alcohol and the essential oils will bead up and when shaken, the liquid clouds up (and eventually separates again).

WHAT YOU WILL NEED:
  2-ounce spray bottle
  1/6 cup perfumer's alcohol – 65% of total amount
  ½ ounce (15ml) distilled water (or hydrosol) – 25% of total amount
  30-60 drops glycerin or base oil – up to 5% of total amount
  30-60 drops essential oil blend – up to 5% of total amount

WHAT TO DO:
1. Fill a clean spray bottle about ½ full with perfume alcohol.

2. Before add all your essential oils, you might want to test your blend. To begin, choose two to three essential oils. Using a dropper, add a total of 10 drops into a small vial. Be sure to write down the number of drops of each oil used (for instance, 5 drops of lemon, 2 drops of lavender, and 3 drops of frankincense). Roll the bottle between your palms to blend oils. Drip your perfume strip in or add a drop to the tip of a perfume strip and sniff to see if you like how your scent has developed. Check your scent again in an hour or two and then again the next day to experience the fragrance's arc.

3. In a separate bowl, add approximately 15-30 drops of your essential oil blend for every ounce of liquid. Add equal amounts of glycerin or base oil. Stir to mix the oils and glycerin completely.

4. Add essential oil blend to the spray bottle then, fill the remaining space with alcohol. Replace cap. Shake to mix.

5. Let the fragrance sit for a couple of weeks in a dark place. Shake bottle everyday to mix contents. Check fragrance after a few weeks to see if ready. Use as normal.

6. You may substitute another liquid for water – perhaps hydrosol, to make your fragrance last longer. Hydrosols, or floral waters are the byproduct from essential oil distillation and contain about 10% essential oil in them. These alone make wonderful body sprays, but can greatly enhance your fragrance blend. Hydrosols add a subtle smell to your spray and are great for the skin. In addition, hydrosols can extend your product's shelf life. Keep in mind recipes that call for products made with water are not for commercial use without the proper use of preservatives to prevent spoilage.

7. Adding glycerin to your body spray is optional, but serves to help moisturize the skin and bring your essential oils together which also helps to hold the fragrance against your skin, making its scent last longer. Jojoba, almond, or olive oil can also be substituted in place of glycerin.

SWEET TARZ
20 drops Orange essential oil
30 drops Cardamom essential oil
10 drops Ginger essential oil

CITRUS BLISS
40 drops Neroli essential oil
20 drops Sandalwood essential oil

SUMMER RAIN
40 drops Spearmint essential oil
20 drops Ylang Ylang essential oil

TROPICAL SEA
20 drops Lime essential oil
20 drops Grapefruit essential oil
20 drops Black Pepper essential oil

ROYAL PRINCE
15 drops Cedarwood essential oil
30 drops Geranium essential oil
15 drops Ginger essential oil

MEN'S AFTERSHAVE

Creating a natural aftershave for someone special is a great way to personalize a blend they can enjoy. This recipe uses a 3% concentration of essential oils and other ingredients (some recipes used Bay Rum). For recipes that are alcohol-based, these are intended for home use only, as special licensing is required for reselling commercial products that contain alcohol. Please check with your local and/state licensing regulations for more information regarding this.

WHAT YOU WILL NEED:
    2-ounce Dark Glass bottle
    Glass Stir Rod
    2-3 tablespoons Alcohol – 94% of total amount
    36 drops Glycerin or Base oil – 3% of total amount
    36 drops Essential oil blend – 3% of total amount

WHAT TO DO:
1. In a small glass bowl, add up to 36 drops of essential oil (or accords) starting with your base note, followed by your middle note, and then top note. You will want to check the fragrance as you add each drop, stirring with a glass rod to blend. Some of the most popular essential oils for men's aftershave include, Bay, Carrot, Roman Chamomile, Cypress, Frankincense, Juniper Berry, Palmarosa, Patchouli, Rosemary, Tea Tree, Sage, and Vetiver.

2. Add in your base oil and/or glycerin. If you do not have glycerin to use as a fixative (which holds the scent to the skin longer), you may use another aloe vera or fractionated coconut oil instead.

3. Add your blend to a dark, glass bottle. Fill the rest of the space with alcohol.

4. Replace cap and shake to blend mixture. Use as normal.

BRAWNY MAN
Basil essential oil
Fir Balsam essential oil
Helichrysum essential oil

CONFIDENT MAN
Cardamom essential oil
Vetiver essential oil
Ylang Ylang essential oil

INSPIRED
Balsam Fir essential oil
Sweet Orange essential oil
Frankincense essential oil

KONA MAN
Black Pepper essential oil
Coriander essential oil
Sandalwood essential oil

TRIATHLON MAN
Cedarwood essential oil
Bergamot essential oil
Sandalwood essential oil

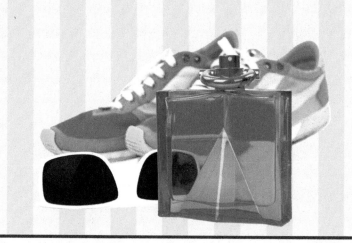

SOOTHING MEN'S AFTERSHAVE (NON-ALCOHOLIC)

For men with sensitive skin or for those times when nicks and cuts, abrasions, or damage skin prevails, try making one of these super nourishing recipes that will moisturize the skin. With these alcohol-free aftershave recipes you can avoid excess drying and irritation and soothe sensitive skin.

WHAT YOU WILL NEED:
> 2-ounce Glass spray bottle
> 2 tablespoons Sweet Almond oil
> 1 tablespoon Aloe Vera Juice
> 12 drops Palmarosa essential oil
> 12 drops Patchouli essential oil
> 12 drops Neroli essential oil
> Distilled Water (as needed)

WHAT TO DO:

1. In a small glass bowl, combine oils, juice and essential oils. Stir to completely blend.

2. Using a funnel, add liquid to glass spray bottle.

3. Add water as needed to thin. Replace cap and shake to blend.

4. Use as needed.

INVIGORATING MEN'S AFTERSHAVE
(NON-ALCOHOLIC)

For men with sensitive skin or for those times when nicks and cuts, abrasions, or damage skin prevails, try making one of these super nourishing recipes that will moisturize the skin. With these alcohol-free aftershave recipes you can avoid excess drying and irritation and soothe sensitive skin.

WHAT YOU WILL NEED:
    2-ounce Glass spray bottle
    ¼ cup Coconut oil
    12 drops Tea Tree essential oil
    12 drops Eucalytpus essential oil
    12 drops Juniper Berry essential oil
    Distilled Water (as needed)

WHAT TO DO:
1. In a small glass bowl, combine oils. Stir to completely blend.

2. Using a funnel, add oils to the glass spray bottle.

3. Add water to thin, if needed.

4. Use as normal.

CLEANSING MEN'S AFTERSHAVE (NON-ALCOHOLIC)

This aftershave recipe offers a combination of healing properties: witch hazel for its astringent effects and jojoba oil delivers hydration to the skin without leaving a greasy residue.

WHAT YOU WILL NEED:
  2-ounce Glass spray bottle
  1/8 cup Jojoba oil
  1/8 cup Witch Hazel
  18 drops Frankincense essential oil
  18 drops Roman Chamomile essential oil
  2-3 drops Vitamin E (as a preservative)
  Glycerin (optional, if needed as a fixative)

WHAT TO DO:
1. In a small glass bowl, combine oils and witch hazel. Add 2-3 drops of Vitamin E oil. Stir to blend well. Add glycerin if needed to help with blending.

2. Using a funnel, add oils to the glass spray bottle. Replace cap and shake to mix.

3. Add distilled water if mixture is too thick to spray. Use as normal.

Rubbing alcohol, Vodka, and Witch Hazel are not suitable substitutions for Perfumer's Alcohol. These are not recommended for using when creating perfume products as they will separate from your essential oils and sometimes cause your perfume to look cloudy.

BASIC PARFUM ROLL-ON RECIPE

Roll-ons are super convenient to carry in your purse and apply on the run! In this recipe, the perfume concentration is 20% (60 drops approximately), but you can add more to your liking. These make wonderful gifts for family and friends.

WHAT YOU WILL NEED:
  15-ml. Glass Roll-On Bottle
  18 drops Top Note Accord
  18 drops Middle Note Accord
  24 drops Base Note Accord
  1 tsp. Fractionated Coconut Oil (or another carrier oil)

WHAT TO DO:
1. In a small glass bowl or shot glass, add your essential oils starting with your middle heart note accord, followed by your base note accord. Make sure these meld together well. Finally, add your top note accords.
2. Remove the roller ball from the bottle.
3. Once you are satisfied with the blend, using a glass dropper, add the oils to the roll-on bottle. Top off with the carrier oil.
4. Replace ball and lid. Shake and roll between the palms to mix thoroughly.
5. Add a decorative label with the name and date created. Use as needed by rolling over pulse points.

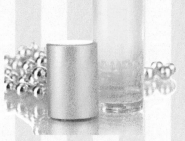

BASIC SOLID PERFUME RECIPE

Making solid perfumes are easy and fun to make. This recipe calls for 40% concentration of oils (approximately 40-50 drops) from all three notes. You may need to double your top note if necessary, since these seem to fade away in the base oil magically. Add more drops for a stronger scent or less for a more subtle fragrance. You can also try two-scent duos such as sweet orange and ylang ylang, cypress and rose, or basil and lime.

WHAT YOU WILL NEED:
    16+ drops Top Note or Accord(s)
    12 drops Middle Note or Accord(s)
    12 drops Base Note or Accord(s)
    ½ tsp. (1/4 oz.) Jojoba or Fractionated Coconut Oil
    ½ tsp. Beeswax Pellets
    Small Tins or Containers

WHAT TO DO:
1. Using a clean, small glass bowl or shot glass, add your accords, starting with the base note, then middle and finally top notes. Be sure to stir as you go, checking the scent.
2. In a double boiler, melt the beeswax pellets on low heat. Once they start to melt, add in the fractionated coconut oil or another carrier oil. You will use equal parts of beeswax to carrier oil.
3. Remove from heat and quickly add your essential oils to the mixture. Stir well.
4. Pour mixture into small tins or containers quickly before it begins to cool and harden. If the wax solidifies, simply pour mixture back into the double boiler to reheat and try again. Don't leave on the stove too long, as the essential oils could evaporate.
5. Within minutes your product will set and will have the consistency of lip balm. Once the solution has hardened (about ten minutes) you can cover and use as needed.

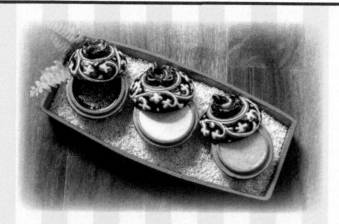

6. Add a label to your product with its name and date.
   Tip: Do not cook the essential oils with the hot wax. This will destroy your essential oils.

Some formulas call for 80% of your favorite carrier oil, 13% beeswax, and 7% of your perfume blend. Others recommend using equal parts of beeswax and carrier oil like this recipe. Trial and error is the best way to determine how much you will need of each. When formulating for a solid perfume, you may want to start with 25% essences, and you can go as high as 40%.

BASIC PERFUME RECIPE (ALCOHOL-BASED)

In this basic recipe, you will be using 40:30:30 proportions for your top, middle, and base notes or accords for your fragrance. Alcohol-based perfumes tend to highlight top note accords, so you will want to adjust the ratio of essences to reach optimal performance. Balancing out the middle and base notes will be necessary for making sure the perfume has the proper sillage. The percentage of essential oil concentration to alcohol ranges from 8-15% for spray perfumes and 18-25% for dab-on perfumes. This one calls for 15% (approximately 90 drops).

WHAT YOU WILL NEED:
    36 drops Top Note Accord(s)
    27 drops Middle Note Accord(s)
    27 drops Base Note Accord(s)
    1 oz. Perfumer's Alcohol
    1 oz. Dark Glass Bottle

WHAT TO DO:
1. In a small glass bowl, add your middle heart note or accord, followed by adding your top note accord. Mix well, smelling and checking the scent. Once you are satisfied with scent, use a glass dropper and funnel to add to the bottle.
2. Fill the remainder of the bottle with the alcohol. Replace top and shake to mix.
3. Allow cologne to sit for fragrances to marry and meld together. It is best to leave for a minimum of six months to mature the composition. Although, if in a hurry, one to two days will work.
4. Once it is ready, you may want to run the liquid through a unbleached coffee filter several times to remove any sediments.
5. Rebottle for storage or place in a beautiful pump-spray bottle ready for use.
    Tip: For dab-on perfumes, you will want to use a higher

concentration of essential oils. Make sure you have enough base notes to keep the fragrance long-lasting, with plenty of heart and top notes that lift around the wearer, making a stunning aura or sillage.

BASIC COLOGNE RECIPE

In this simple recipe, you will be using only top and middle notes for your perfume. The percentage of your essential oil concentration to alcohol range from 2-4%. This one is using 3% (approximately 18 drops). You could use vodka instead of perfumer's alcohol if its only for personal use.

WHAT YOU WILL NEED:
>   16 drops Top Note Accord(s)
>   2 drops Middle Note Accord(s)
>   1 oz. Perfumer's Alcohol
>   1 oz. Dark Glass Bottle

WHAT TO DO:
1. In a small glass bowl, add your heart note or accord, followed by adding your top note accord. Mix well, smelling and checking the scent. Once you are satisfied with the scent, use a glass dropper and funnel to add to the bottle.
2. Fill the remainder of the bottle with the alcohol. Replace top and shake to mix.
3. Allow cologne to sit for fragrances to marry and meld together. It is best to leave for a minimum of six months to mature the composition. Although, if in a hurry, one to two days will work.
4. Once it is ready, you may want to run the liquid through a unbleached coffee filter several times to remove any sediments.
5. Rebottle for storage or place in a beautiful pump-spray bottle ready for use.

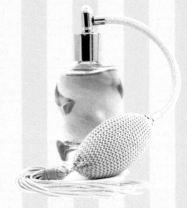

BASIC PERFUME ROOM SPRAY RECIPE

Here's an easy room spray recipe you can make in just minutes. Using a room spray is an excellent way to freshen your surroundings and brighten things up. Not only will the essential oils make your space smell great, but you will also be reaping the health benefits of the essential oils as well. The possibilities for this room spray recipe are endless!

WHAT YOU WILL NEED:
  4 oz. Hydrosol, Floral Water, or Distilled Water
  1 tbsp. Glycerin (as a fixative)
  18-30 drops Top Note Essential Oil or Accord
  12-20 drops Middle Note Essential Oil or Accord
  6-10 drops Base Note Essential Oil or Accord
  4oz Glass or Plastic Spray Bottle

WHAT TO DO:
1. In a clean spray bottle, add the fixative (Glycerin, or Witch Hazel if making a facial spray).
2. Add your essential oil to the fixative, starting with the base note, followed by the middle note, and then the top note. Shake well.
3. Pour the hydrosol or floral water into the bottle and shake to mix contents well.
4. If you want to make this a facial spray instead, use three ounces of hydrosol with one-ounce of witch hazel.
   Tip: If using around children or pets, please check precautions for the essential oils you choose.

BASIC PERFUME OIL RECIPE

Whether it's soft and subtle or exotic and romantic, you can quickly make any fragrance you desire. This basic recipe can be changed and adapted to your own signature style, depending on what you like. Keep track of what you add or change, so you'll know how to make your favorite blends at a later time. This recipe uses the blending by note 3-2-1 method. However, if you prefer another method, you will want to use a 15-30% concentration.

WHAT YOU WILL NEED:
    ½ oz. Jojoba Oil (or another favorite carrier oil)
    30 drops Vitamin E Oil
    15 drops Top Note Essential Oil
    10 drops Middle Note Essential Oil
    5 drops Base Note Essential Oil
    1 oz. Dark Bottle

WHAT TO DO:
1. Add your carrier oil such as jojoba to a clean, dark glass bottle.
2. In a separate bowl, add Vitamin E oil (10%) and 30 drops of your perfume blend (10%). Mix well, and add to the bottle.
3. When adding essential oils or accords separately, start with the base note and add the middle note, followed by the top note. As you add each one, check the scent to make sure it is what you are looking for.
4. Allow your perfume to sit for 48 hours up to six weeks. The longer it sits, the stronger the fragrance will intensify.
5. Remove the cap and see if it has the desired scent you are looking for. If not, you can add more essential oils and let it sit longer until you get the desired scent.
6. At the end of this maturing process, your perfume should be ready. Store your perfume in a cool, dark place. Don't forget to name your creation!

Tip: You will have to play around with scents for a little bit before you hit on what you like. Make sure that you write each ratio of every essential oil used in a particular scent as nothing can be more frustrating than actually coming up with the fragrance of your dreams and then not remembering how you ended up making it.

BASIC PERFUME OIL RECIPE #2

This basic recipe uses the 40:30:30 ratio of notes at 30% concentration, which of course you can change and adapt to your own preference. Make sure to write down what you add or change, so you'll remember how you made it.

WHAT YOU WILL NEED:
　　½ oz. Jojoba Oil (or another favorite carrier oil)
　　36 drops Top Note Essential Oil or Accord
　　27 drops Middle Note Essential Oil or Accord
　　27 drops Base Note Essential Oil or Accord
　　1 oz. Dark Bottle

WHAT TO DO:
1. Add your carrier oil such as jojoba to a clean, dark glass bottle.
2. In a separate bowl, add 90 drops of your perfume blend (30%). Mix well, and add to the bottle.
3. When adding each accord, start with the heart note, then add the base note next, followed by the top note accord. As you add each one, check the scent to make sure it is pleasing.
4. Allow your perfume to sit for 48 hours up to six weeks. The longer it sits, the stronger the fragrance will intensify.
5. Remove the cap and see if it has the desired scent you are looking for. If not, you can add more essential oils and let it sit longer until you get the desired scent.
6. At the end of this maturing process, your perfume should be ready. Store your perfume in a cool, dark place. Don't forget to label your bottle with its name and date you made it.

BASIC PERFUME BODY OIL RECIPE

Here is an easy-to-follow basic recipe for making body oil or massage blends! You get to decide which essential oils to use depending on the type of massage and affect you looking to achieve.

WHAT YOU WILL NEED:
　　1 oz. (30 ml.) Carrier Oil, Lotion, or Gel
　　9-15 drops Top Note Essential Oil
　　6-10 drops Middle Note Essential Oil
　　3-5 drops Base Note Essential Oil
　　1 oz. Plastic Bottle

WHAT TO DO:
1. Pour your carrier oil, lotion or gel into a clean bottle.
2. Add your essential oils one drop at a time, starting with your base note, followed by the middle note, and then the top note.
3. Shake well to mix oils and carrier together.
4. Add a label with name, ingredients, and date created.
5. Use as normal.

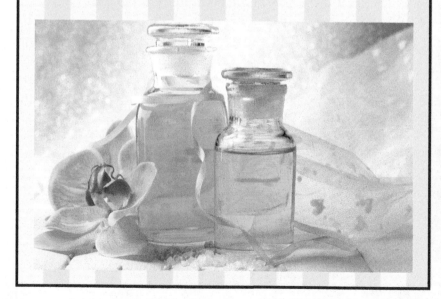

BASIC PERFUME LINEN SPRAY RECIPE

Use this unique blend for helping with insomnia or to freshen your bed linens. Don't forget when using essential oils for your spray to take into consideration whether they are stimulating or relaxing!

WHAT YOU WILL NEED:
   8 oz. Hydrosol or Floral Water (or Distilled Water)
   1 tbsp. Glycerin
   60 drops Top Note Essential Oil
   40 drops Middle Note Essential Oil
   20 drops Base Note Essential Oil
   8 oz. Glass or Plastic Spray Bottle

WHAT TO DO:
   1. In a clean spray bottle, add the fixative (glycerin).
   2. Add your essential oil to the fixative, starting with the base note, followed by the middle note, and then the top note. Shake well.
   3. Pour the hydrosol or floral water into the bottle and shake to mix contents well.
   4. Spray on bedspread and linens before making the bed.

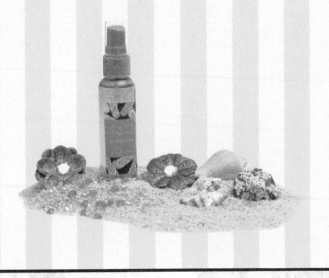

BASIC PERFUME BODY LOTION RECIPE

Do you want to try a good body lotion recipe? Why not make your own today by following these simple instructions?

WHAT YOU WILL NEED:
   4 oz. Unscented Lotion, Carrier Oil or Hydrosol
   18 drops Top Note Essential Oil
   12 drops Middle Note Essential Oil
   6 drops Base Note Essential Oil
   4 oz. Plastic Bottle or Container

WHAT TO DO:
   1. Place your carrier oil and/or lotion in your bottle.
   2. Add essential oils starting with your base note essential oil first, followed by the middle note, and then the top note essential oil.
   3. Recap and shake well to mix.
   4. Use as normal.

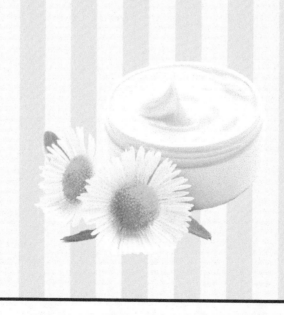

BASIC RECIPES

ENDNOTES

1. http://www.naturalperfumers.com/definition.php
2. http://www aftelier.com/Essence-Alchemy-p/wb-book-essencealchemy.htm
3. http://www.pourlemondeparfums.com/naturalvssynthetic.html
4. "Natural Perfume vs. Synthetic Perfume." Pour le Monde Parfums, http://www.pourlemondeparfums.com/naturalvssynthetic.html
5. Source: http://www.naturalperfumers.com/definition.php
6. http://essentialoilsacademy.com
7. http://www.webmd.com/allergies/features/fragrance-allergies-a-sensory-assault
8. http://askjan.org/media/fragrance.html
9. http://www.everydayhealth.com/allergies/fragrance-sensitivity.aspx
10. Michael Edwards, Fragrances of the World. Sydney: Michael Edwards & Co., 2008

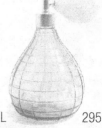

ENDNOTES

APPENDIX A

DILUTION RATE FOR FORMULAS

Use this chart as a quick guide for each product type. The difference is simply the amount of oils in each product. Keep in mind these are general guidelines for determining concentrations. You may want to use more or less. They are as follows: perfume (15-40%), eau de perfume (10-15%), eau de toilette (5-15%), cologne (1-3%), and room sprays (1-5%).

PRODUCT	ESSENTIAL OILS %	PERFUMER'S ALCOHOL %	WATER %
Perfume	15 - 40	65 - 85	0 - 10
Eau de perfume	10 - 15	75 - 90	0 - 10
Eau de toilette	5 - 15	65 - 85	10 - 20
Eau de cologne	3 - 5	65 - 70	25 - 30
Cologne	1 - 3	77 - 80	15 - 20
Room Spray	1 - 5	75 - 80	20

APPENDICES

APPENDIX B
AN OVERVIEW OF THE MAIN MATERIAL
GROUPS USED IN THE PERFUME INDUSTRY

A liquid that is made from a mixture of various aroma materials of natural and/or synthetic origin is known as a PERFUME CONCENTRATE, popularly known as the "COMPOUND" in the fragrance industry.

The different aroma materials that are used in making perfumes are described below. The percentage of each aroma material reflects the proportion of that material that may be present in modern perfumes. However, purely natural perfumes are available as well, and the percentages will be different based on the materials used.

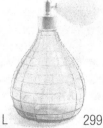

Essential Oils & Extracts – 0-30%

Steam Or Water/Steam Distilled

The plant cells are ruptured by the steam, and the volatile oil that is present in the cells is vaporized. Using the distillation process, the steam is then cooled to form water. The volatile oil either floats on the surface of water or sinks at the bottom, thereby, getting separated.

The essential oils that are produced by this method are usually of a light color because the color molecules are typically non-volatile and large in size.

Flowers from which the oil is extracted by steam:

  Lavender
  Ylang ylang

Leaves from which the oil is extracted by steam:

  Eucalyptus
  Geranium

Buds/Seeds from which the oil is extracted using steam:

  Clove
  Cardamom

Grasses from which the oil is extracted using steam:

  Vetiver
  Lemongrass

Woods from which the oil is extracted using steam:

  Turpentine
  Sandalwood

Expressed from citrus fruits

The oil is present in the tiny translucent sacs found in the skin of the fruit, which is expressed by squeezing. The oil is then separated from the juice of the fruit. The oils expressed from the citrus fruits are usually of a lighter color than the color of the fruit they are obtained from.

Fruits from which the oil is expressed by squeezing:

  Orange
  Lemon

Extracted

The plant is treated with a solvent such as hexane, petroleum ether or cyclohexane, which dissolves the wax, oil, and color from the plant. CONCRETE is then produced by evaporating the solvent. Alcohol is used to remove the wax present in the concrete. Alcohol is then evaporated leaving a dark colored ABSOLUTE.

Flowers from which the oil is extracted using a solvent:

  Jasmine
  Rose

Gums from which the oil is extracted using solvents:

  Benzoin
  Labdanum

Lichens from which the oil is extracted using solvents:

  Oakmoss
  Treemoss

Animal Products – 0-0.1%

Tinctures: The glands of animals or their secretions are dissolved in alcohol. The alcohol is then evaporated to produce a dark colored ABSOLUTE.

Musk is obtained from Tibetan Deer

Castoreum is derived from Beaver

Civet is obtained from Cat

Ambergris is obtained from Whale

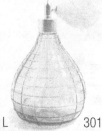

Aroma Chemicals - 70-100%

Crude Oil Isolates

Raw chemicals, which are not added in perfumes including Toluene, Benzene, Naphthalene, Xylol and Phenol, are obtained from crude oil. These compounds then go through a series of complex reactions to form numerous synthetic aroma chemicals. These chemicals are sometimes referred to as Nature Identical as many of them resemble the chemicals found in nature.

Aroma chemicals which are obtained from Benzene:

  P.E.A.
  Galaxolide

Aroma chemicals which are obtained from Toluene:

  Benzyl
  Acetate

Aroma chemicals which are obtained from Naphthalene:

  Methyl
  Anthranilate

Aroma chemicals which are obtained from Phenol:

  Eugenol
  Evernyl

Aroma chemicals which are obtained from Xylene:

  Musk Xylol
  Musk Ketone

Essential Oil Isolates

A single chemical that is separated from any essential oil is referred to as essential oil isolates. They may be produced by physical means such as distillation or cooling, in which case they are referred to as natural chemicals. These chemicals are very often used either as a starting material in a long series of complex reaction or to make numerous other chemicals by simple reactions including acetylation.

Aroma chemicals which are obtained from Turpentine:

  Pinene
  (Linalool)

Aroma chemicals which are obtained from Lemongrass:

  Citral
  (Ionone)

Aroma chemicals which are obtained from Clove:

  Eugenol
  (Vanillin)

Aroma chemicals which are obtained from Vetiver:

  Vetiverol
  (Vetiveryl Acetate)

Aroma chemicals which are obtained from Peppermint:

  Menthol
  (Menthyl Acetate)

APPENDIX C

COMPANION OIL CHART

Use this chart as a guide for finding essential oils that complement one another in a blend.

ESSENTIAL OIL	COMPANION OILS
Ajowan (Bishop's Weed)	Parsley, Sage, Thyme
Allspice	Bay, Black Pepper, Cistus Labdanum, Coriander, Geranium, Ginger, Lavender, Neroli, Opoponax, Orange, Patchouli, Ylang Ylang
Ambrette Seed	Clary Sage, Cypress, Frankincense, Neroli, Patchouli, Rose, Sandalwood
Amyris	Cedarwood, Citronella, Ginger, Ho Wood, Lavender, Oakmoss, Balsam Peru, Ylang Ylang
Angelica Root	Bergamot, Clary Sage, Eucalyptus, Frankincense, Grapefruit, Juniper Berry, Lemon, Lemongrass, Lime, Oakmoss, Opoponax, Orange, Patchouli, Rosemary, Vetiver
Angelica Seed	Bergamot, Cardamom, Clary Sage, Coriander, Fennel, Geranium, Jasmine, Lemon, Rose, Sage
Aniseed	Bay, Cinnamon, Clove Bud, Fennel, Frankincense, Geranium, Ginger, Grapefruit, Lavender, Lemon, Mandarin, Myrrh, Peppermint, Pine, Orange, Spearmint
Anise Star	Bay, Cardamom, Caraway Seed†, Cedarwood, Coriander, Fennel, Galbanum, Lavender, Mandarin, Orange, Pine, Rose, spice oils
Balsam, Fir	Benzoin, Cedarwood, Cypress, Juniper Berry, Pine, Sandalwood, other balsams
Balsam, Copaiba	Cananga, Cedarwood, Clary Sage, Frankincense, Jasmine, Rose, Sandalwood, Vanilla, Violet, Ylang Ylang, citrus oils, spice oils, floral oils
Balsam, Gurjun	Ambrette Seed
Balsam, Peru	Cardamom, Cinnamon, Clove Bud, Coriander, Grapefruit, Mandarin, Patchouli, Petitgrain, Orange, Rose, Sandalwood, Tuberose, Ylang Ylang, spice oils, floral oils
Balsam, Poplar	German Chamomile, Helichrysum, Yarrow, spice oils, floral oils
Balsam, Tolu	Cedarwood, Cistus Labdanum, Neroli, Sandalwood, Ylang Ylang, spice oils, floral oils

ESSENTIAL OIL	COMPANION OILS
Basil, Sweet*	Bergamot, Black Pepper*, Cedarwood, Citronella, Clary Sage, Coriander, Cypress, Fennel, Geranium, Hyssop, Lavender, Ginger, Grapefruit, Jasmine, Lemon, Lime, Marjoram, Neroli, Niaouli, Oakmoss, Opoponax, Orange, Palmarosa, Pine, Rosemary, Sage, Tea Tree, Thyme, Vetiver
Bay Laurel	Benzoin, Bergamot, Black Pepper, Cardamom, Cinnamon, Clary Sage, Clove Bud, Cistus Labdanum, Coriander, Cypress, Frankincense, Geranium, Ginger, Grapefruit, Juniper Berry, Lavender, Lemon, Mandarin, Orange, Patchouli, Pine, Rosemary, Sage†, Ylang Ylang, citrus oils
Bay, West Indies	Bergamot, Black Pepper, Cardamom, Cinnamon, Clove Bud, Coriander, Frankincense, Geranium, Ginger, Grapefruit, Lavender, Lavandin, Lemon, Mandarin, Nutmeg, Orange, Petitgrain, Rosemary, Sandalwood, Ylang Ylang
Benzoin	Bay, Bergamot, Black Pepper, Balsam Copaiba, Cardamom, Coriander, Cypress, Frankincense, Ginger, Geranium, Grapefruit, Jasmine, Juniper Berry, Lemon, May Chang, Myrrh, Nutmeg, Orange, Rose, Sandalwood, Ylang Ylang
Bergamot	Black Pepper, Chamomile, Clary Sage, Coriander, Cypress, Frankincense, Geranium, Helichrysum, Jasmine, Juniper Berry, Lavender, Mandarin, Melissa, Neroli, Nutmeg, Orange, Rose, Sandalwood, Vetiver, Violet, Ylang Ylang
Bitter Orange	Bay, Black Pepper, Cinnamon, Clove Bud, Clary Sage, Cypress, Frankincense, Ginger, Grapefruit, Lavender, Lemon, Lime, Myrrh, Myrtle, Neroli, Petitgrain, Vetiver
Birch	Balsam Fir, Black Pepper, Cinnamon, Cedarwood, Clove Bud, Balsam Copaiba, Eucalyptus, Frankincense, Patchouli, Myrrh, Myrtle, Sandalwood, Spruce, Rosemary, Rosewood, Thyme, Vetiver, woody oils
Black Pepper*	Bergamot, Cardamom, Clary Sage, Clove Bud, Coriander, Fennel, Frankincense, Geranium, Ginger, Grapefruit, Juniper Berry, Lavender, Lemon, Lemongrass, Lime, Mandarin, Marjoram, Myrrh, Orange, Nutmeg, Palmarosa, Rose, Rosemary, Sage, Sandalwood, Tea Tree, Vetiver, Ylang Ylang
Blue Tansy	Cedarwood, Lavender, Helichrysum, Pine, Ravensara, Rosemary
Cajeput	Bergamot, Birch, Cardamom, Clary Sage, Clove Bud, Geranium, Lavender, Marjoram, Myrtle, Nutmeg*, Oakmoss, Pine, Rose, Rosemary, Thyme, spice oils, Ylang Ylang

ESSENTIAL OIL	COMPANION OILS
Camphor, White*	Black Pepper, Cardamom, Eucalyptus, Frankincense, Lavender, Lemon, Marjoram, Mandarin, Orange, Peppermint, Ravensara, Rosemary, Spearmint, Tea Tree, Thyme, Yarrow, Ylang Ylang, citrus oils, spice oils
Cananga	Bergamot, Birch, Balsam Copaiba, Jasmine, Cistus Labdanum, Lavender, Lemon, Neroli, Oakmoss, Palmarosa, Sandalwood, Vetiver, Ylang Ylang
Caraway Seed*	Basil, Bay, Black Pepper, Chamomile, Cinnamon Leaf, Coriander, Cassia†, Eucalyptus, Frankincense, Galbanum, Ginger, Jasmine, Lavender, Mandarin, Orange, Rosemary, Tangerine, spice oils
Cardamom	Bay, Bergamot, Black Pepper, Caraway Seed†, Cedarwood, Cinnamon Leaf, Clove Bud, Coriander, Fennel, Frankincense, Galbanum, Geranium, Ginger, Grapefruit, Jasmine, Juniper Berry, Labdanum, Lemon, Lemongrass, Mandarin, May Chang, Myrtle, Neroli, Orange, Palmarosa, Patchouli, Petitgrain, Rose, Sandalwood, Vetiver, Ylang Ylang
Carrot Seed	Bergamot, Cedarwood, Cinnamon Geranium, Juniper Berry, Lavender, Lemon, Lime, Mimosa, Neroli, Orange, Petitgrain, Rosemary, citrus oils, spice oils
Cassia	Black Pepper, Coriander, Frankincense, Ginger, Geranium, Rosemary, citrus oils
Catnip	Grapefruit, Lavender, Lemon, Marjoram, Peppermint, Orange, Rosemary, Spearmint
Celery Seed	Black Pepper, Coriander, Ginger, Lavender, Lovage, Oakmoss, Opoponax, Pine, Tea Tree
Cedarwood, Atlas	Bay, Bergamot, Cardamom, Roman Chamomile, Cistus Labdanum, Clary Sage, Cypress, Eucalyptus, Fir, Frankincense, Jasmine, Juniper Berry, Lavender, Mandarin, Orange, Neroli, Palmarosa, Petitgrain, Pine, Rosemary, Rosewood, Sandalwood, Vetiver, Ylang Ylang, floral oils
Cedarwood, Texas	Patchouli, Pine, Spruce, Vetiver
Cedarwood, Virginian	Benzoin, Bergamot, Cinnamon, Cypress, Frankincense, Jasmine, Juniper Berry, Lavender, Lemon, Neroli, Patchouli, Rose, Rosemary, Sage, Sandalwood, Vetiver
Cedar Leaf (Thuja)	Bergamot, Cedarwood, Lavender, Pine Needle, Sandalwood, citrus oils
Cedar, Western Red	Bergamot, Benzoin, Cypress, Cinnamon, Frankincense, Juniper Berry, Jasmine, Lemon, Lime, Lavender, Rose, Neroli, Rosemary

ESSENTIAL OIL	COMPANION OILS
Chamomile, German	Benzoin, Bergamot, Roman Chamomile, Cistus Labdanum, Clary Sage, Cypress, Frankincense, Geranium, Grapefruit, Jasmine, Lavender, Lemon, Marjoram, Neroli, Niaouli, Patchouli, Pine, Ravensara, Rose, Rosemary, Sage, Tea Tree, Ylang Ylang, citrus oils
Chamomile, Maroc	Bay, Benzoin, Bergamot, Cardamom, Cedarwood, Coriander, Cypress, Frankincense, Geranium, Grapefruit, Lavender, Lemon, Lemongrass, Mandarin, Marjoram, Oakmoss, Orange, Patchouli, Petitgrain, Vetiver, Ylang Ylang
Chamomile, Roman	Bergamot, Clary Sage, Cistus Labdanum, Eucalyptus, Galbanum, Geranium, Grapefruit, Jasmine, Lavender, Lemon, Neroli, Palmarosa, Oakmoss, Rose, Rosemary, Tea Tree
Cinnamon Bark	Bay, Balsam Peru, Benzoin, Bergamot, Cardamom, Cedarwood, Clove Bud, Coriander, Frankincense, Geranium, Ginger, Grapefruit, Lavender, Lemon, Lemongrass, Mandarin, Marjoram, Nutmeg, Neroli, Palmarosa, Patchouli, Peppermint, Petitgrain, Orange, Vanilla, Ylang Ylang
Cinnamon Leaf	Bay, Balsam Peru, Benzoin, Bergamot, Caraway Seed†, Cardamom, Clove Bud, Coriander, Frankincense, Geranium, Ginger, Grapefruit, Lemon, Lemongrass, Mandarin, Marjoram, Myrtle, Nutmeg*, Orange, Patchouli, Peppermint, Petitgrain, Rose, Vanilla, Ylang Ylang, citrus oils
Cistus Labdanum	Bergamot, Cedarwood, Roman Chamomile, Clary Sage, Cypress, Frankincense, Galbanum, Jasmine, Juniper Berry, Lavender, Lemon, Lime, Myrrh, Nutmeg, Oakmoss, Opoponax, Orange, Patchouli, Pine, Rose, Sandalwood, Spearmint, Vetiver
Citronella	Bergamot, Cedarwood, Geranium, Lemon, Orange, Pine, Sandalwood
Clary Sage	Bay, Bergamot, Black Pepper, Cardamom, Cedarwood, German Chamomile, Roman Chamomile, Coriander, Cypress, Frankincense, Geranium, Grapefruit, Jasmine, Juniper Berry, Lavender, Lemon, Lime, Mandarin, Melissa, Neroli, Patchouli, Petitgrain, Pine, Orange, Rose, Rosewood, Sandalwood, Tea Tree, Ylang Ylang
Clove Bud	Allspice, Bay, Basil, Benzoin, Bergamot, Black Pepper*, Cananga, Roman Chamomile, Cinnamon Leaf, Citronella, Clary Sage, Geranium, Ginger, Grapefruit, Jasmine, Lavandin, Lavender, Lemon, Mandarin, Nutmeg*, Orange, Palmarosa, Peppermint, Rosemary, Rose, Sandalwood, Vanilla, Ylang Ylang

ESSENTIAL OIL	COMPANION OILS
Coriander	Bergamot, Black Pepper*, Cardamom, Cinnamon Leaf, Citronella, Clary Sage, Clove Bud, Cypress, Frankincense, Galbanum, Geranium, Ginger, Grapefruit, Jasmine, Lemon, Neroli, Nutmeg, Orange, Palmarosa, Petitgrain, Pine, Ravensara, Sandalwood, Vetiver, Ylang Ylang, spice oils
Cumin	Cardamom, Galbanum, Lavandin, Lavender, Rosemary, Rosewood
Cypress	Ambrette, Benzoin, Bergamot, Black Pepper, Cardamom, Cedarwood, Cistus Labdanum, Clary Sage, Clove Bud, Cypress, Eucalyptus, Frankincense, Geranium, Ginger, Grapefruit, Jasmine, Juniper Berry, Lavender, Lemon, Lime, Mandarin, Marjoram, Moroccan Chamomile, Neroli, Nutmeg, Orange, Pine, Ravensara, Rosemary, Sandalwood, citrus oils
Cypress, Blue	Cardamom, Cedarwood, Clary Sage, Jasmine, Juniper Berry, Lavender, Lemon Myrtle, Geranium, Orange, Pine, Rose, Sandalwood, Tea Tree
Davana	Amyris, Bergamot, Black Pepper, Cardamom, Roman Chamomile, Jasmine, Mandarin, Neroli, Orange, Patchouli, Rose, Rosewood, Sandalwood, Spikenard, Tangerine, Tuberose, Vanilla, Ylang Ylang
Dill	Aniseed, Bay, Bergamot, Black Pepper, Caraway Seed†, Cardamom, Cinnamon, Clove Bud, Coriander, Elemi, Fennel, Geranium, Ginger, Juniper, Lemon, Mandarin, Nutmeg*, Orange, Peppermint, Pimento Berry, Spearmint, spice oils, citrus oils
Douglas Fir	German Chamomile, Cedarwood, Cistus Labdanum, Cypress, Fir Needle, Frankincense, Juniper Berry, Lavender, Lemon, Marjoram, Myrtle, Pine, Sandalwood, Rosemary, Rosewood
Elemi	Bay, Benzoin, Cinnamon Leaf, Cistus Labdanum, Clove Bud, Frankincense, Ginger, Hyssop, Lavandin, Lavender, Lemon, Lemongrass, Marjoram, Myrrh, Orange, Petitgrain, Rosemary, Sage†, Sandalwood, spice oils
Eucalyptus Globulus	Cedarwood, German Chamomile, Roman Chamomile, Coriander, Cypress, Juniper Berry, Lavender, Lemon, Lemongrass, Marjoram, Peppermint, Pine, Rosemary, Thyme
Eucalyptus Citriodora	Basil, Black Pepper, Cedarwood, Clary Sage, Clove Bud, Cypress, Eucalyptus, Frankincense, Geranium, Ginger, Juniper Berry, Lavender, Marjoram, Orange, Peppermint, Pine, Ravensara, Rosemary, Sage, Tea Tree, Thyme, Vetiver, Ylang Ylang

ESSENTIAL OIL	COMPANION OILS
Eucalyptus Dives	Aniseed, Basil, Cajeput, Cedarwood, Citronella, Frankincense, Ginger, Hyssop, Juniper Berry, Lavender, Lemon, Marjoram, Myrtle, Niaouli, Pine, Peppermint, Rosemary, Spearmint, Tea Tree, Thyme
Eucalyptus Polybractea	Angelica Root, Aniseed, Basil, Cajeput, Cedarwood, Citronella, Frankincense, Ginger, Hyssop, Juniper Berry, Lavender, Lemon, Marjoram, Myrtle, Niaouli, Pine, Peppermint, Rosemary, Spearmint, Tea Tree, Thyme
Eucalyptus Radiata	Basil, Camphor, German Chamomile, Cypress, Fir, Frankincense, Geranium, Ginger, Grapefruit, Helichrysum, Hyssop, Juniper, Lavender, Lemon, Lemongrass, Melissa, Myrtle, Peppermint, Pine, Rosemary, Sandalwood, Tea Tree, Thyme
Fennel	Basil, Bergamot, Black Pepper, Cardamom, Coriander, Cypress, Dill, Fir, Geranium, Ginger, Grapefruit, Juniper Berry, Lavender, Lemon, Mandarin, Marjoram, Niaouli, Orange, Peppermint, Pine, Ravensara, Rose, Rosemary, Sandalwood, Spearmint, Tangerine, Ylang Ylang
Fir (Silver Fir or Fir Needle)	Benzoin, Cistus Labdanum, Galbanum, Lavender, Lemon, Marjoram, Orange, Pine, Rosemary
Fir Balsam	Benzoin, Cistus Labdanum, Clary Sage, Ginger, Lavender, Marjoram, Pine, Rosemary, citrus oils
Fir, White	Basil, Bergamot, Benzoin, Birch, Camphor, Cedarwood, Cistus Labdanum, Clary Sage, Cypress, Frankincense, Geranium, Ginger, Hyssop, Lavender, Lemon, Marjoram, Myrtle, Orange, Pine, Rosemary, Thyme, citrus oils
Fleabane	Cardamom, Cilantro, Coriander, citrus oils
Frankincense	Basil, Bergamot, Black Pepper*, Cinnamon Leaf, Cypress, Galbanum, Geranium, Grapefruit, Lavender, Lemon, Mandarin, Neroli, Orange, Palmarosa, Patchouli, Pine, Rose, Sandalwood, Vetiver, White Camphor, Ylang Ylang
Galbanum	Benzoin, Bergamot, Clary Sage, Cedarwood, Maroc Chamomile, Cinnamon, Citronella, Clove Bud, Coriander, Cypress, Elemi, Fir, Frankincense, Geranium, Ginger, Grapefruit, Jasmine, Lavender, Lemon, Lemongrass, Linden Blossom, Myrrh, Oakmoss, Opoponax, Orange, Palmarosa, Patchouli, Pine, Rose, Sandalwood, Spruce, Styrax, Tuberose, Vetiver, Violet, Ylang Ylang
Garlic	None known

ESSENTIAL OIL	COMPANION OILS
Geranium	Benzoin, Bergamot, Black Pepper, Cedarwood, Roman Chamomile, Citronella, Clary Sage, Clove Bud, Cypress, Fennel, Frankincense, Ginger, Grapefruit, Jasmine, Juniper Berry, Lavender, Lemon, Lime, Mandarin, Neroli, Orange, Palmarosa, Patchouli, Peppermint, Petitgrain, Rose, Rosemary, Sandalwood, Ylang Ylang
Ginger	Bergamot, Cedarwood, Cinnamon Leaf, Coriander, Clove Bud, Coriander, Elemi, Eucalyptus, Frankincense, Geranium, Grapefruit, Jasmine, Juniper Berry, Lemon, Lime, Mandarin, Myrtle, Neroli, Orange, Palmarosa, Patchouli, Rose, Rosemary, Rosewood, Sandalwood, Spearmint, Vetiver, Ylang Ylang
Goldenrod	Balsam Peru, Ginger, Spruce
Grapefruit	Bergamot, Black Pepper, Cardamom, Clary Sage, Clove Bud, Cypress, Eucalyptus, Fennel, Frankincense, Geranium, Ginger, Juniper Berry, Lavender, Lemon, Mandarin, Neroli, Oakmoss, Palmarosa, Patchouli, Peppermint, Orange, Rose, Rosemary, Sandalwood, Thyme, Ylang Ylang, citrus oils, floral oils, spice oils
Helichrysum (italicum)	Bergamot, Black Pepper, Cedarwood, German Chamomile, Clary Sage, Clove Bud, Cypress, Frankincense, Geranium, Grapefruit, Juniper Berry, Lavender, Lemon, Mandarin, Neroli, Oakmoss, Oregano, Palmarosa, Pine, Rose, Rosemary, Sage, Tea Tree, Thyme, Vetiver, Ylang Ylang, citrus oils
Helichrysum (odoratissimum)	Bergamot, German Chamomile, Clary Sage, Clove Bud, Geranium, Labdanum, Lavender, Oakmoss, Balsam Peru, Rose, citrus oils
Ho Wood	Basil, Cajeput, Chamomile, Lavender, Sandalwood, Ylang Ylang
Holy Basil	Bergamot, Clary Sage, Geranium, Hyssop, Lime, Sweet Myrrh, Oakmoss, Citronella
Hyssop	Bay, Bay Laurel, Bergamot, Cedarwood, Celery, Clary Sage, Cypress, Eucalyptus, Frankincense, Fennel, Geranium, Grapefruit, Lavender, Lemon, Mandarin, Marjoram, Myrrh, Myrtle, Orange, Rosemary, Sage†, citrus oils
Inula	Rosalina
Jasmine	Bay, Benzoin, Bergamot, Clary Sage, Clove Bud, Coriander, Geranium, Ginger, Grapefruit, Lemon, Mandarin, Neroli, Orange, Palmarosa, Patchouli, Petitgrain, Rose, Sandalwood, Ylang Ylang, floral oils, citrus oils

ESSENTIAL OIL	COMPANION OILS
Juniper Berry	Benzoin, Bergamot, Black Pepper, Cedarwood, Cistus Labdanum, Clary Sage, Cypress, Elemi, Eucalyptus, Fennel, Fir Needle, Frankincense, Galbanum, Geranium, Grapefruit, Lavandin, Lavender, Lemon, Mandarin, Oakmoss, Pine, Rosemary, Sage, Sandalwood, Balsam Tolu, Vetiver, citrus oils
Lavandin	Bay Laurel, Bergamot, Cinnamon Leaf, Citronella, Clary Sage, Clove Bud, Cinnamon Leaf, Cypress, Geranium, Lime, Patchouli, Pine, Rosemary, Thyme, citrus oils
Lavender, Spike	Angelica Root, Aniseed, Bay Laurel, Bergamot, Black Pepper, Cinnamon Leaf, Citronella, Clary Sage, Clove Bud, Cinnamon Leaf, Cypress, Geranium, Lime, Patchouli, Pine, Rosemary, Thyme, citrus oils
Lavender, True	Angelica Root, Aniseed, Bergamot, Black Pepper, Camphor, Cedarwood, German Chamomile, Roman Chamomile, Clary Sage, Clove Bud, Cypress, Eucalyptus, Geranium, Grapefruit, Juniper Berry, Cistus Labdanum, Lemon, Lemongrass, Mandarin, Marjoram, Oakmoss, Palmarosa, Patchouli, Peppermint, Pine, Ravensara, Rose, Rosemary, Tea Tree, Thyme, Vetiver, citrus oils, floral oils
Lemon	Basil, Bay, Benzoin, Bergamot, Roman Chamomile, Citronella, Cistus Labdanum, Clary Sage, Dill, Elemi, Eucalyptus, Fennel, Frankincense, Galbanum, Geranium, Hyssop, Juniper Berry, Lavandin, Lavender, Neroli, Nutmeg, Oakmoss, Orange, Peppermint, Rose, Rosemary, Sandalwood, Violet, Ylang Ylang, citrus oils
Lemongrass	Basil, Bay, Bergamot, Black Pepper, Cardamom, Cedarwood, Cinnamon Bark, Clary Sage, Clove Bud, Coriander, Cypress, Frankincense, Fennel, Geranium, Ginger, Grapefruit, Hyssop, Lavender, Lemon, Jasmine, Mandarin, Marjoram, Nutmeg, Orange, Palmarosa, Patchouli, Petitgrain, Rosemary, Spikenard, Tea Tree, Thyme, Vetiver, Yarrow, Ylang Ylang
Lime	Citronella, Clary Sage, Lavandin, Lavender, Neroli, Nutmeg, Rosemary, Vanilla, Ylang Ylang, citrus oils
Linaloe Berry	Cedarwood, Frankincense, Rose, Rosewood, Sandalwood, woody oils, floral oils
Linden Blossom	Black Pepper, Clove Bud, Frankincense, Geranium, Jasmine, Lemon, Mandarin, Neroli, Orange, Petitgrain, Rose, Sandalwood, Tuberose, Ylang Ylang
Lovage Leaf	Bay, Galbanum, Lavender, Oakmoss, Opoponax, Rose, spice oils

ESSENTIAL OIL	COMPANION OILS
Mandarin	Basil, Bergamot, Black Pepper, Roman Chamomile, Cinnamon Bark, Clove Bud, Clary Sage, Frankincense, Geranium, Grapefruit, Jasmine, Juniper Berry, Lavender, Lemon, Lime, Neroli, Orange, Palmarosa, Patchouli, Petitgrain, Rose, Sandalwood, Ylang Ylang, spice oils
Marjoram, Sweet	Basil, Bergamot, Black Pepper, Cedarwood, Roman Chamomile, German Chamomile, Clary Sage, Cypress, Eucalyptus, Fennel, Juniper Berry, Lavender, Lemon, Mandarin, Orange, Nutmeg*, Peppermint, Pine, Rosemary, Tea Tree, Thyme, Ylang Ylang
May Chang	Basil, Bay, Black Pepper, Cardamom, Cedarwood, Roman Chamomile, Clary Sage, Coriander, Cypress, Eucalyptus, Frankincense, Geranium, Ginger, Grapefruit, Juniper Berry, Marjoram, Orange, Palmarosa, Patchouli, Petitgrain, Rosemary, Sandalwood, Tea Tree, Thyme, Vetiver, Ylang Ylang
Melaleuca (Tea Tree)	Cananga, Clary Sage, Clove Bud, Geranium, Lavandin, Lavender, Marjoram, Nutmeg*, Oakmoss, Pine, Rosemary, spice oils
Melissa (Lemon Balm)	Roman Chamomile, Frankincense, Geranium, Lavender, Neroli, Petitgrain, Rose, citrus oils
Mugwort (Wormwood)	Aniseed, Angelica, Lavender, Orange, Jasmine, Oakmoss
Myrrh	Bergamot, Benzoin, German Chamomile, Clove Bud, Cypress, Eucalyptus, Frankincense, Galbanum, Geranium, Grapefruit, Hyssop, Juniper Berry, Lavender, Lemon, Mandarin, Oakmoss, Palmarosa, Patchouli, Pine, Rosemary, Sandalwood, Thyme, Ylang Ylang, mint oils, spice oils
Myrtle	Basil, Bay, Bay Laurel, Benzoin, Bergamot, Cardamom, Cinnamon Leaf, Clary Sage, Clove Bud, Coriander, Eucalyptus, Galbanum, Geranium, Ginger, Helichrysum, Hyssop, Lavandin, Lavender, Lemon, Lemongrass, Lime, Mandarin, Orange, Rosemary, Spearmint, Tea Tree, Thyme, spice oils
Neroli	Benzoin, Roman Chamomile, Coriander, Frankincense, Geranium, Grapefruit, Jasmine, Juniper Berry, Lemon, Mandarin, Myrrh, Orange, Petitgrain, Rose, Sandalwood, Ylang Ylang, citrus oils
Niaouli	Basil, Cajeput, Eucalyptus, Fennel, Juniper Berry, Lavender, Lemon, Lime, Myrtle, Orange, Pine, Rosemary, Peppermint, Tea Tree, Thyme
Nutmeg	Bay, Bay Laurel, Cinnamon Bark, Clove Bud, Coriander, Clary Sage, Geranium, Jasmine, Lavandin, Lemon, Lime, Mandarin, Oakmoss, Orange, Peru Balsam, Petitgrain, Rose, Rosemary, spice oils

ESSENTIAL OIL	COMPANION OILS
Oakmoss	Amyris, Angelica, Basil, Cananga, Celery, Galbanum, Grapefruit, Juniper Berry, Cistus Labdanum, Lavender, Lemon, Lovage, Tagetes, Moroccan Chamomile, Myrrh, Nutmeg*, Oregano†, Palmarosa, Patchouli, Roman Chamomile, Sandalwood, Spikenard, Spruce, Summer Savory†, Tarragon, Tea Tree, Valerian, Vetiver, Yarrow
Opoponax	Bergamot, Clary Sage, Coriander, Fir Needle, Frankincense, Cistus Labdanum, Myrrh, Neroli, Patchouli, Sandalwood, Vetiver
Orange, Blood	Bay, Bergamot, Clary Sage, Clove Bud, Lavender, Lemon, Myrrh, Nutmeg
Orange, Sweet	Bay, Benzoin, Bergamot, Black Pepper, Cinnamon Leaf, Clary Sage, Clove Bud, Coriander, Frankincense, Geranium, Ginger, Grapefruit, Jasmine, Juniper Berry, Lavender, Lemon, May Chang, Marjoram, Myrrh, Neroli, Nutmeg*, Patchouli, Petitgrain, Rose, Sandalwood, Vetiver, Ylang Ylang
Oregano, Common	Cedarwood, Citronella, Lavandin, Oakmoss, Pine, Rosemary, Lavender, White Camphor
Oregano, Spanish	Cedarwood, German Chamomile, Cypress, Eucalyptus, Lavender, Mandarin, Orange, Nutmeg*, Rosemary, Thyme, Ylang Ylang
Palmarosa	Amyris, Bay, Benzoin, Bergamot, Cananga, Cedarwood, Roman Chamomile, Clary Sage, Clove Bud, Coriander, Frankincense, Geranium, Ginger, Grapefruit, Juniper Berry, Lemon, Lemongrass, Mandarin, Oakmoss, Orange, Patchouli, Petitgrain, Rose, Rosemary, Rosewood, Sandalwood, Ylang Ylang, floral oils
Palo Santo	Cedarwood, Sandalwood, woody oils
Patchouli	Bergamot, Black Pepper, Cedarwood, Cinnamon, Cistus Labdanum, Clary Sage, Clove Bud, Coriander, Frankincense, Geranium, Ginger, Grapefruit, Jasmine, Lavender, Lemongrass, May Chang, Mandarin, Myrrh, Neroli, Oakmoss, Orange, Rose, Sandalwood, Vetiver, Ylang Ylang
Peppermint	Basil, Benzoin, Bergamot, Black Pepper, Cypress, Eucalyptus, Geranium, Grapefruit, Juniper Berry, Lavender, Lemon, Marjoram, Niaouli, Pine, Ravensara, Rosemary, Sandalwood, Spearmint, Tea Tree, Wintergreen
Petitgrain	Basil, Benzoin, Bergamot, Cedarwood, Clary Sage, Clove Bud, Cypress, Eucalyptus, Frankincense, Geranium, Jasmine, Juniper Berry, Lavender, Lemon, Mandarin, Marjoram, Neroli, Orange, Palmarosa, Patchouli, Rose, Rosemary, Sandalwood, Ylang Ylang, citrus oils

ESSENTIAL OIL	COMPANION OILS
Pimento Leaf	Bay, Bergamot, Camphor, Cinnamon Leaf, Clove Bud, Frankincense, Ginger, Geranium, Jasmine, Lavender, Lemon, Mandarin, Orange, Patchouli, Petitgrain, Rose, Ylang Ylang
Pine, Long Leaf	Bergamot, White Camphor, Cedarwood, Citronella, Clary Sage, Cypress, Eucalyptus, Fir Needle, Frankincense, Grapefruit, Juniper Berry, Lavender, Lemon, Marjoram, Peppermint, Oakmoss, Pine, Ravensara, Rosemary, Sandalwood, Tea Tree, Thyme
Pine, Scotch	Bergamot, Cedarwood, Citronella, Clary Sage, Cypress, Eucalyptus, Juniper Berry, Lavender, Lemon, Marjoram, Niaouli, Rosemary, Sage†, Tea Tree
Plai	Black Pepper, Lavender, Neroli, Orange, Rosemary, Sandalwood
Ravensara	Clove Bud, Eucalyptus, Lavender, Rosemary.
Ravintsara	Basil, Cedarwood, Cinnamon Leaf, Clove Bud, Eucalyptus, Lavender, Marjoram, Oregano, Peppermint, Pine, Rosemary, Sandalwood
Rosalina	Cypress, Lemon, Myrtle, Tea Tree, Peppermint
Rose Otto	Balsam Peru, Benzoin, Bergamot, Roman Chamomile, Clary Sage, Clove Bud, Geranium, Jasmine, Lavender, Lemon, Mandarin, Neroli, Palmarosa, Petitgrain, Sandalwood, Ylang Ylang
Rosemary	Basil, Bergamot, Black Pepper, Cedarwood, Cinnamon Leaf, Cistus Labdanum, Citronella, Clary Sage, Cypress, Elemi, Eucalyptus, Frankincense, Geranium, Grapefruit, Juniper Berry, Lavender, Lavandin, Lemon, May Chang, Mandarin, Marjoram, Niaouli, Oregano, Palmarosa, Peppermint, Petitgrain, Pine, Ravensara, Tea Tree, Thyme, Rose, spice oils
Rosewood	Floral oils, spice oils, wood oils
Sage	Basil, Cedarwood, Maroc Chamomile, Cypress, Hyssop, Lavandin, Lavender, Lemon, Myrtle, Orange, Peppermint, Petitgrain, Pine, Rosemary, Rosewood, Thyme, Yarrow, citrus oils
Sandalwood	Benzoin, Bergamot, Black Pepper*, Roman Chamomile, Clary Sage, Clove Bud, Fennel, Frankincense, Geranium, Grapefruit, Jasmine, Labdanum, Lavender, Lemon, Mandarin, Myrrh, Neroli, Oakmoss, Orange, Palmarosa, Patchouli, Petitgrain, Rose, Rosewood, Tuberose, Vetiver, Violet, Ylang Ylang
Savory, Wild	Citrus oils, Lavender, Oakmoss, Pine, Rosemary
Spearmint	Basil, Bergamot, Eucalyptus, Jasmine, Lavandin, Lavender, Peppermint, Rosemary, Sandalwood

ESSENTIAL OIL	COMPANION OILS
Spikenard	Clary Sage, Clove Bud, Cistus Labdanum, Cypress, Fir Needle, Frankincense, Geranium, Juniper Berry, Lavender, Lemon, Myrrh, Neroli, Oakmoss, Palmarosa, Patchouli, Pine, Rose, Vetiver, spice oils
Spruce, Black	Benzoin, Cedarwood, Galbanum, Lavandin, Lavender, Oakmoss, Pine, Rosemary
Styrax	Bay, Cardamom, Cinnamon Bark, Clove Bud, Geranium, Ginger, Helichrysum, Jasmine, Lavender, Lemon, Nutmeg, Orange, Rose, Violet, Ylang Ylang, spice oils
Tagetes	Clary Sage, Jasmine, Lavender, Bergamot, citrus oils
Tangerine	Basil, Bergamot, Cinnamon Leaf, Clary Sage, Clove Bud, Frankincense, Lavender, Lemon, Lime, Neroli, Orange
Tansy, Blue	Pine, Cedarwood, Lavender, Rosemary, Ravensara, Helichrysum
Tarragon*	Basil, Bergamot, Roman Chamomile, Clary Sage, Frankincense, Galbanum, Geranium, Grapefruit, Cistus Labdanum, Lavender, Lemon, Lime, Neroli, Oakmoss, Orange, Pine, Rose, Vanilla
Thyme	Peru Balsam, Bergamot, Birch, Clary Sage, Cypress, Eucalyptus, Frankincense, Geranium, Ginger, Grapefruit, Hyssop, Lemon, Lavender, Lavandin, Mandarin, Marjoram, Melissa, Myrtle, Orange, Palmarosa, Pimento Berry, Pine, Rosemary
Tsuga (Hemlock)	Amyris, Benzoin, Clary Sage, Pine, Cedarwood, Galbanum, Lavender, Oakmoss and Rosemary
Tuberose	Balsam Peru, Benzoin, Bergamot, Jasmine, Mandarin, Orange, Rose, Sandalwood
Turmeric	Cananga, Clary Sage, Ginger, Cistus Labdanum, Orris
Valerian	Cedarwood, Lavender, Mandarin, Oakmoss, Patchouli, Petitgrain, Pine, Rosemary
Vanilla	Balsams, Benzoin, Opoponax, Sandalwood, Vetiver, spice oils
Verbena, Lemon	Basil, Bergamot, Geranium, Lemon, Elemi, Neroli, Palmarosa, Rosemary
Vetiver	Bergamot, Black Pepper, Clary Sage, Coriander, Eucalyptus, Geranium, Ginger, Grapefruit, Jasmine, Lavender, Lemon, Lemongrass, May Chang, Mandarin, Melissa, Oakmoss, Opoponax, Orange, Patchouli, Rose, Sandalwood, Violet, Ylang Ylang

ESSENTIAL OIL	COMPANION OILS
Violet Leaf	Basil, Bay, Cinnamon Leaf, Clary Sage, Clove Bud, Cumin, Geranium, Grapefruit, Hop, Jasmine, Lavender, Lemon, Rose, Sandalwood, Tangerine, Tarragon, Tuberose, floral oils
White Lotus	Floral oils
Wintergreen	Birch, Lavender, Marjoram, Peppermint, Ylang Ylang, Vanilla
Yarrow	Bergamot, Birch, Black Pepper, Cedarwood, Roman Chamomile, Clary Sage, Cypress, Eucalyptus, Fennel, Frankincense, Geranium, Ginger, Helichrysum, Lavender, Lemon, Marjoram, Myrtle, Oakmoss, Peppermint, Pine, Rosemary, Sage, Valerian, Vetiver
Ylang Ylang	Balsam Peru, Bergamot, Roman Chamomile, Clary Sage, Clove Bud, Eucalyptus, Ginger, Grapefruit, Jasmine, Lavender, Lemon, May Chang, Mandarin, Neroli, Opoponax, Orange, Palmarosa, Patchouli, Petitgrain, Rose, Rosewood, Sandalwood, Tuberose, Vetiver

† Toxic. Do not use on skin. *Use in small quantities.

APPENDICES

APPENDIX D
SOURCE GUIDE

You will need a variety of supplies ranging from funnels to beakers for measuring, blending, and bottles and containers for storing your custom blends, essential oils, and alcohol. Numerous suppliers offer quality products at a reasonable price. Here are a few of the top suppliers to choose from.

AROMATHERAPY CERTIFICATION TRAINING

AROMA HUT INSTITUTE
Aromatherapy Certification Program and Essential Oil Classes; Franchises available to graduates.
HTTP://AROMAHUT.COM

PROFESSIONAL INSURANCE

INDIE BEAUTY NETWORK
HTTP://WWW.INDIEBEAUTY.COM
Offers insurance for aromatherapy companies and a network for finding businesses and advertising.

BOTTLES

SKS BOTTLE & PACKAGING, INC.
A varied selection of glass and plastic bottles, jars, lip balm tubes, and more.
Phone: 518-880-6980
Fax: 518-880-6990
WWW.SKS-BOTTLE.COM

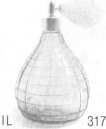

E.D. LUCE PACKAGING
Unique bottles: lip balm, roll-on perfume, small frosted sprays, and perfume bottles, and more.
Phone: 562-802-0515
Fax: 562-802-0501
WWW.ESSENTIALSUPPLIES.COM

SPECIALTY BOTTLES
A varied selection of glass and plastic bottles and jars.
Phone: 206-340-0459
WWW.SPECIALTYBOTTLES.COM

BEST BOTTLES
They are a distributor of glass bottles for perfume, decorative glass containers, atomizers, sprayers, roll-on bottles, perfume vials, droppers, funnels and more.
HTTP://WWW.BESTBOTTLES.COM

GSZ CORPORATION
Unique Czech Bohemian Glass Perfume oil bottles.
HTTP://WWW.GSZCORPORATION.COM/PERFUME_BOTTLES1.HTM

ESSENTIAL OILS

HEAL WITH OIL
WWW.HEALWITHOIL.COM
Wholesale program with 100% pure therapeutic grade quality essential oils.

CAMDEN GREY
Perfume Strips ($24 for 500)
HTTP://WWW.CAMDENGREY.COM/ESSENTIAL-OILS/PERFUMERY-TESTERS/PERFUME-TEST-STRIP.HTML

VETIVER AROMATICS
An international supplier of resources and information for making perfume. All of their oils are phthalate free and vegan. They also offer complete perfume-making kits, perfume strips, and more. They supply materials and ingredients to customers in North America, Europe, Australia, Africa, and India.
HTTP://VETIVERAROMATICS.COM/
Phone: 812-518-2173

CARRIERS

THE JOJOBA COMPANY
Unrefined, organic Jojoba Oil in bulk.
Phone: 800-256-5622
WWW.JOJOBACOMPANY.COM

NEW DIRECTIONS AROMATICS INTERNATIONAL
Pure essential oils, fragrance oils, and carrier oils.
WWW.NEWDIRECTIONSAROMATICS.COM

UNSCENTED LOTION/MASK

ELIZABETH VAN BUREN, INC.
Unscented aroma lotion and masks.
Phone: 800-710-7759
WWW.ELIZABETHVANBUREN.COM

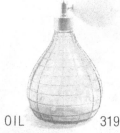

GLASS STIR RODS AND POURING BEAKERS

INDIGO INSTRUMENTS
WWW.INDIGO.COM

SCIENCE LAB
HTTP://WWW.SCIENCELAB.COM/PAGE/S/PVAR/22-1900

ACCESSORIES FOR FRAGRANCES
Provides supplies including atomizers, roll-ons, glass vials, perfume bottles, funnels, pipettes and much more for perfume-making.
WWW.ACCESSORIESFORFRAGRANCES.COM

SAVE ON SCENTS
Producer of fragrance oils and craft supplies.
HTTP://WWW.SAVEONSCENTS.COM

SUNROSE AROMATICS
Provider of essential oils and plant aromatics.
HTTP://WWW.SUNROSEAROMATICS.COM

WATERPROOF LABELS
Online Labels – Provider of labels all shapes and sizes; thousands of choices.
WWW.ONLINELABELS.COM

PLASTIC PIPETTES
Rachel's Supply – Provider of various supplies, including plastic pipettes.
WWW.RACHELSUPPLY.COM

EUROPEAN COMMISSION
Pharmaceuticals and Cosmetics; INCI labeling information.
HTTP://EC.EUROPA.EU/GROWTH/SECTORS/COSMETICS/INDEX_EN.HTM

INTERNATIONAL FRAGRANCE ASSOCIATION
Information regarding the manufacturing and handling of fragrance materials. A voluntary code of practice governs the use of aroma materials in perfumery.
HTTP://WWW.IFRAORG.ORG/EN/INGREDIENTS

UNITED STATES FDA COSMETIC WEBSITE
Cosmetic information regarding its uses.
HTTP://WWW.FDA.GOV/COSMETICS/DEFAULT.HTM

FDA PRODUCT DEFINITIONS & INFORMATION
Guidelines and Regulatory Information.
HTTP://WWW.FDA.GOV/COSMETICS/
GUIDANCECOMPLIANCEREGULATORYINFORMATION/UCM074201.HTM

FDA VOLUNTARY COSMETIC REGISTRATION PROGRAM
Registration program.
HTTP://WWW.FDA.GOV/COSMETICS/
GUIDANCECOMPLIANCEREGULATORYINFORMATION/
VOLUNTARYCOSMETICSREGISTRATIONPROGRAMVCRP/DEFAULT.HTM

FDA COSMETIC LABELING AND LABELING CLAIMS
How to properly label ingredients.
HTTP://WWW.FDA.GOV/COSMETICS/COSMETICLABELINGLABELCLAIMS/DEFAULT.
HTM

ALCOHOL AND TOBACCO TAX AND TRADE BUREAU
Laws and regulations regarding denatured alcohol use.
HTTP://WWW.TTB.GOV/INDUSTRIAL/SDA.SHTML

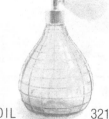

NATURAL PERFUMERS GUILD

The only international trade organization dedicated to promoting the beauty and benefits of 100% natural fragrances and giving a voice to the artisan natural perfumer.

HTTP://WWW.NATURALPERFUMERS.COM

INDEPENDENT PERFUMERS GUILD

IPG's primary goals are to promote handmade artisan fragrances. Free to join.

HTTP://INDIEPERFUMERSGUILD.TUMBLR.COM/

NATURAL PERFUMERY

HTTPS://GROUPS.YAHOO.COM/NEO/GROUPS/NATURALPERFUMERY/INFO

APPENDIX E

ODOR INTENSITY CHART

As you will discover, some essential oils have a stronger odor potency than others. In order to prevent having one oil overpower your blend, you may choose to use less of that oil for that note. Professional perfumers use an odor intensity chart as a quick reference when determining which oils work well together in an accord.

Become familiar with your oils by writing down a number between 1 and 10, based on your own interpretation of its intensity. Several have been filled in already to help you get started, but feel free to change its odor intensity classification if you consider a particular oil to be more or less powerful.

The odor intensity scale for each oil is from 1 to 10.
    1 = Most Strong. Use less in a formula.
    10 = Very volatile and light. Use more in a formula.

HOW TO DETERMINE AN OIL'S ODOR INTENSITY

Begin by taking out two oils of the same note you want to work with. Dip a clean perfume strip into the first oil and wave beneath your nose. Now, take another clean perfume strip and dip the strip into the second oil and wave beneath your nose. Which one smells stronger to you? Write the name of each oil on its strip and place the least intense oil strip down on the table. Now, take another oil out of the same note, and repeat this procedure again comparing it to the first oil that was considered more intense. Mark and place the strip down that is less intense next to the first oil. If you consider the third oil to be more intense than the strip on the table, you can change the order of your strips on the table based on intensity. Once you have compared all of your oils from one note classification (Top, Middle, or Base) and have them laid out in order by intensity, fill in this chart with its odor intensity factor you determined. Do this for the oils you have on hand or as you begin to work through your collection. Have your coffee beans on hand and take breaks as needed.

Ajowan		Fleabane		Petitgrain	
Allspice		Frankincense	7	Pimento Leaf	
Angelica Root		Galbanum		Pine	
Aniseed		Garlic		Plai	
Ambrette Seed		Geranium	6	Ravensara	
Balsam		Ginger	6	Ravintsara	
Anise Star		Gingergrass		Rosalina	
Balsam Fir		Goldenrod		Rose	7
Benzoin	4	Grapefruit	4	Rose Geranium	
Basil		Helichrysum	7	Rosemary	
Bay		Ho Wood		Rosewood	5
Bay Laurel		Hyssop		Sage	
Black Pepper	7	Inula		Sandalwood	5
Bergamot	4	Jasmine	7	Scotch Pine	
Birch		Juniper Berry	5	Spearmint	
Blue Tansy		Lavandin		Spikenard	
Cajeput		Lavender	5	Spruce	
Camphor		Lemon		Tagetes	
Cananga		Lemon Myrtle		Tangerine	
Caraway Seed		Lemongrass		Tarragon	
Cardamom		Lime		Tea Tree	
Carrot Seed		Linaloe Berry		Thyme	
Cassia		Mandarin		Tulsi	
Cedar Leaf		Marjoram	5	Turmeric	
Cedarwood	4	May Chang		Valerian	
Chamomile	8	Melissa		Vanilla	
Cinnamon	6	Myrrh	7	Verbena	
Cistus Labdanum		Myrtle		Vetiver	9
Citronella		Neroli	5	Violet Leaf	
Clary Sage	5	Niaouli		Wild Tansy	
Clove Bud	8	Nutmeg		Winter Savory	
Coriander		Oakmoss		Wintergreen	
Cumin		Opoponax		Wormwood	
Cypress	4	Orange, Bitter		Ylang Ylang	6
Davana		Orange, Sweet	4	Yarrow	
Dill		Oregano		Xanthoxylum	
Douglas Fir		Palmarosa	5		
Elemi		Palo Santo			
Eucalyptus	8	Parsley			
Fennel	6	Patchouli	6		
Fir Needle		Peppermint	7		

APPENDIX F
GLOSSARY OF TERMS

ABSORPTION RATE
The rate at which an essential oil or carrier oil penetrates the skin over a given period of time (can be subjective).

ABSOLUTE
A concentrated, highly aromatic, oily mixture extracted from plants using solvent extraction techniques producing a waxy mass called concrete. The lower molecular weight, aromatic compounds are extracted from the concrete into ethanol. When the ethanol evaporates, the absolute is left behind.

ACCORD
A blend of two or more fragrances that combine to produce a new, entirely different odor impression.

ADULTERATE
To make impure by adding extraneous, improper, or inferior ingredients.

ALCOHOL
The word used by itself usually refers to Ethyl Alcohol or Ethanol, the main solvent used to carry perfume for extracts or colognes. When referring to its chemical name, it refers to the chemical group R-OH.

ALDEHYDE
Organic compounds present in many natural materials and are synthesized artificially. This refers to the chemical group R-CHO. The word by itself usually refers to shorter (C6-C12) straight chain (aliphatic) aldehydes used in perfumery. Chanel No. 5 is an aldehydic floral perfume.

ALLERGY
A hypersensitivity to certain substances such as pollens, foods, or microorganisms, which cause an overreaction of the immune system with symptoms such as a skin rash, swelling of mucous membranes, sneezing or wheezing, or other abnormal conditions.

ANIMALIC
Animal-derived ingredients such as civet, ambergris, musk, and castoreum. Usually reproduced synthetically in modern perfumery. Often strong and unpleasant in their concentrated form, in smaller amounts these notes provide depth to a fragrance.

ANOSMIC
Having no sense of smell.

ANTI-ALLERGENIC
A substance capable of preventing an allergic reaction.

APOCRINE SWEAT GLANDS
The glands on the human body that give you your unique scent, which can interfere with or enhance the scent of perfumes you wear.

AROMA CHEMICALS
Chemicals that have a smell and/or taste that are used in perfumes or flavors. Note: the term "aromatic chemicals" should not be confused as it refers to the Benzene ring structure found in many organic compounds.

AROMACHOLOGY
The science, coined by the Olfactory Research Fund, dedicated to the study of the interrelationship between psychology and aroma.

AROMATHERAPY
The art and science of using essential oils to heal common ailments and/or complaints. Therapy with aroma can be particularly helpful with stress or emotionally triggered problems such as insomnia and headaches. The term "aromatherapy" was coined by a French chemist, R. M. Gattefosse.

AROMATIC
Refers to the Benzene ring structure found in many organic compounds. However, the term in perfumery refers to the rich aroma displayed by balsamic notes.

ATTAR (OTTO)
From the ancient Persian word "to smell sweet." Attar or Otto refers to essential oil obtained by distillation and, in particular, that of the Bulgarian Rose, an incredibly precious perfumery material.

AQUEOUS
Refers to scents that are based on a concept of a watery smell.

BALANCE
A fragrance that has been carefully crafted and blended so well that it has no one identifiable component, but creates one harmonious effect.

BALSAM
A water soluble, semi-solid or viscous resinous exudates similar to that of gum.

BALSAMIC
Rich, sweet, resinous and warm notes produced by using plant balsams and resins. The oriental fragrance category is characterized by these ingredients.

BASE NOTES
The third and last phase (after top [head] and middle [heart] notes) of a perfume's evaporation, left on the skin.

BODY NOTE
The main characteristic of a note when smelling the oil on a perfume strip.

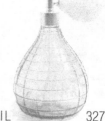

BOTANICAL NAME

A scientific name in Latin that conforms to the International Code of Botanical Nomenclature (ICBN) and is a certain species of plant that clearly distinguishes it from other plants that share the same common name. The purpose of a formal name is to have a single name that is accepted and used worldwide for a particular plant or plant group.

BOUQUET

A mixture of flower notes.

CAMPHORACEOUS

The fresh, clean, cooling character displayed by eucalyptus but also descriptive of rosemary and other herbal notes.

CARRIER OIL

A vegetable fatty oil used to dilute essential oils for the purpose of application to the skin or massage.

CHARACTER

What makes a fragrance, note, or perfume distinct.

CHEMOTYPES

The same botanical species occurring in other forms due to different growth conditions.

CHYPRE

Pronounced "sheepra" and French for cyprus. Refers to woody, mossy, earthy scents.

CITRUS

The fresh, slightly sour notes displayed by lemon, orange, grapefruit, and bergamot.

CO2 EXTRACTS

Oils that are extracted by the carbon dioxide method are commonly referred to as CO2 Extracts or CO2s for short. Essential oils processed by this method are considered superior in that none of the constituents have been harmed by heat, have a closer aroma to the natural source and are generally thicker oils.

COHOBATION

A process in the extraction method of essential oil (especially rose) that ensures it is a complete oil.

COLD-PRESSED

Refers to a method of extraction where no external heat is applied during the process.

COMMON NAME

The everyday name used for a plant. Names such as Chamomile, Lavender, Orange, or Eucalyptus may refer to more than one species, yet go by the same name. It is necessary to know its botanical name for clarity.

COMPOUND

The concentrated fragrance mixture before it is diluted to make the finished perfume. Also called perfume oil.

CONCRETE

A waxy, concentrated, semi-solid essential oil extract made from plant material that is used to make an absolute.

DECOCTION

An herbal preparation made by boiling the plant material and reducing into a concentration.

DEPTH

A fragrance that is rich, full-bodied, and deep.

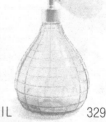

DIFFUSER
A device used to disperse the aromatic molecules of essential oils into the air.

DISCORD
A fragrance that is disjointed and lacks harmony.

DISTILLATE
A product of distillation. For instance, lavender oil is the distillate of the fresh, blooming lavender plant.

DISTILLATION
A method of extraction used in the manufacture of essential oils.

DRAM
A unit of measurement equaling a 1/8 of an ounce.

DRYDOWN
The final phase—or bottom note—of a fragrance, which emerges several hours after application. Perfumers evaluate the base notes and the tenacity of the fragrance during this stage.

EARTHY
Notes that give the impression of earth, soil, the forest floor, mold, and moss.

EAU DE COLOGNE
A solution of about three percent (3%) perfume compound in an alcohol/water base. Much lighter than a concentrated perfume.

EAU DE PARFUM
An alcoholic perfume solution containing ten to fifteen percent (10-15%) perfume compound.

EAU DE TOILETTE
An alcohol/water-based perfume solution containing three to eight percent (3-8%) perfume compound.

EMOLLIENT
A substance that softens and soothes the skin.

ESSENTIAL OIL
An aromatic, volatile liquid consisting of odorous principles from plant extracts.

EVANESCENT
A fleeting or quickly vanishing note or fragrance.

EXPRESSION
An extraction method where plant materials are pressed to obtain the essential oil.

EXTRAIT (EXTRACT)
An alternative name for alcoholic perfumes. Extraits contain fifteen to forty-five percent (15-45%) perfume compound in alcohol.

EXUDATES
A natural substance secreted by plants that can be spontaneous or as a result of damage to the plant.

FIXATIVE
A natural or synthetic substance used to slow down the evaporation of volatile components in a perfume and improve stability when added to more volatile components. This will make your fragrance last longer.

FIXED OILS
Vegetable oils obtained from plants that are fatty and non-volatile.

FLAT
A fragrance that is devoid of interesting qualities and lacks character, diffusiveness, and distinction.

FLORAL
Perfumes characterized by the prevalence of well defined floral notes.

FLORAL-FRUITY
Perfumes having notably fruity elements, generally in the top notes, as an accessory to floral heart notes.

FOLD
Refers to the percentage of terpenes removed by re-distillation from single fold to fivefold.

FOUGÈRE
From the French for fern. Fougère scents are based on a herbaceous accord and may include notes such as lavender, coumarin, oakmoss, woods, and bergamot.

FRACTIONATED OIL
A process in which oils are re-distilled, either to have terpenes or other substances removed.

FULL-BODIED
A fragrance that is rich with a robust scent.

GREEN
The general term for the odors of grass, leaves and stems.

HARMONIOUS
In perfumery, this term is used to describe the final outcome and impression of an accord.

HEADY
An invigorating and exhilarating effect a perfume has. Its odor is considered powerful and intoxicating and stimulates the senses.

HEART (MIDDLE) NOTES
The second phase of a perfume's evaporation on the skin, which gives the scent its character after the top notes fade.

HERBACEOUS
A note that is naturally fresh, leafy or hay-like, such as chamomile or clary sage.

HESPERIDIA
A general term for citrus oils.

HYDRO DIFFUSION
A method of extracting essential oils in which steam at atmospheric pressure is passed through the plant material from the top of the extraction chamber, resulting in oils that retain the original aroma of the plant; this process is less harsh than steam distillation.

HYDROSOL (FLORAL WATER)
The water resulting from the distillation of essential oils, which still contains some of the properties of the plant material from the extraction process.

INFUSED OIL
Oil produced by steeping the macerated botanical material in the liquid until it has taken on some of the plant material's properties.

INFUSION
The process of making an herbal remedy by steeping plant material in water to extract its soluble principles.

IONONES
Highly valued synthetic chemicals, used in small amounts in many floral, green, and woody perfumes. Produces a scent similar to violet or iris.

JUICE
A term used in perfumery referring to the alcoholic solution of the perfume composition.

LIFT
When a citrus or top note is used in a perfume it adds life, brilliance and diffusiveness to a blend. This can be achieved by adding the finished fragrance to a base composition. The perfumer has a repertoire of bases on hand for this purpose.

LEATHER
Pungent animal smokiness characteristic of the ingredients used in tanning leathers. Achieved in perfumery with castoreum, labdanum, and synthetic chemicals.

MACERATE
To make soft by soaking or steeping in a liquid.

MATURATION
The ideal stage of a perfume at the end of the period of maceration.

MOSSY
Fragrances with earthy, aromatic forest scents.

NOSE
A person who mixes fragrance components to make perfume, AKA a perfumer.

OLEORESIN
Natural resinous exudation from plants or aromatic liquid extracted from botanical material.

OLEO GUM RESIN
Odoriferous exudation from botanical material consisting of essential oil, gum, and resin.

OLFACTION
Refers to the sense of smell.

OLFACTORY BULB
The bulblike distal end of the olfactory lobe center where the processing of smell is started and is then passed on to other areas of the brain.

ORGAN
A desk-like unit designed in a semi-circular shape with shelves for holding raw materials for perfumery, such as essential oils, arranged by scent category. A perfumer sits at the organ and can arrange a perfume selecting notes, much like a musician who plays the musical instrument.

ORIENTAL
Fragrance family based on balsamic, exotic aromas such as vanilla, oakmoss, and animal notes. These scents are usually suited to evening wear.

ORIFICE REDUCER
A small plastic insert inside the glass bottle that acts as a dropper. To use, just tip the bottle to count out the number of drops.

OXIDATION
The process of the addition of oxygen to an organic molecule, or the removal of electrons or hydrogen from the molecule.

OZONIC
Aroma chemicals that are meant to mimic the smell of fresh air after a thunderstorm.

PERFUME (EXTRAIT)
The most highly concentrated and longest-lasting form of fragrance, containing between twenty to fifty percent (20-50%) perfume compound.

PHEROMONE
A substance released by an animal that serves to influence the physiology or behavior of other members of the same species, as a chemical messenger sent between two people.

PHYTOHORMONES
Plant substances mimicking the actions of human hormones. Plant hormones in the plant control or regulate germination, growth, metabolism, or other physiological activities.

PIPETTE
A plastic dropper used to dispense essential oil from a bottle into another bottle or container.

POMADE
Perfumed fat obtained during the effleurage extraction method.

POWDERY
A baby-powder scent effect, produced when a heavier, sweet or woody note is blended with a lighter note such as a citrus, fruity or light green note.

RECTIFICATION
A process of re-distilling essential oils to remove certain constituents and purify it.

REPERTOIRE
A collection of finished fragrances used for evaluation, samples, marketing, and sales.

RESIN
A natural substance exuded from trees; prepared resins are oleoresins from which the essential oil has been removed.

RESINOIDS
Perfumed material extracted from natural resinous material by solvent extraction. Extracts of resinous gums, balsams, resins or roots. Commonly used as fixatives in perfume compositions.

RICH
A perfume that possesses fullness, depth and body.

ROUNDED

A perfume that has the finishing touches added and is balanced, smooth, and harmonious.

SHARP

A strong, penetrating, sometimes pungent fragrance.

SHEER

A term used in marketing that describes a polished fragrance.

SHELF LIFE

The amount of time a carrier or base oil will remain fresh before oxidizing and becoming rancid.

SILLAGE

The trail of scent left behind by a perfume. Fragrances with minimal sillage are often said to stay close to the skin like an aura.

SMOOTH

A perfume that is harmonious, balanced and well rounded. The tones are soft, and no harshness is present.

SOLIFLORE

A fragrance that focuses on a single flower.

SPICY

Piquant or pungent notes that have a warm or hot character, such as clove, cinnamon and thyme oil.

STABILITY

Refers to how long a scent lasts, either in the bottle or when exposed to elements such as heat, light, and air.

STRENGTH

The relative intensity of a fragrance impression.

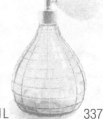

SYNERGY

Several substances or agents working together in harmony to produce a greater effect than the sum of the individual agents. A synergistic blend of essential oils would be one with the correct proportions of oils that have a greater effect than that of an individual oil.

SYNTHETIC

A substance produced by chemical synthesis, especially not of natural origin.

TENACITY

A property of a fragrance whose effect is persistent.

TERPENE

One of a class of hydrocarbons with an empiric formula of C10H16, occurring in essential oils and resins.

TERPENELESS

An essential oil from which monoterpene hydrocarbons have been removed.

THIN

A fragrance lacking the overtones that give it richness and body, or a composition that does not have enough components.

TINCTURE

An alcoholic solution prepared from herbal or perfume material.

TONALITY

The dominant note of a fragrance.

TONE

The tonality or ambience of a fragrance.

TONE DOWN

To reduce the intensity of a note in a composition.

TOP NOTES
The impression of a fragrance when first smelled or applied to the skin. Usually the most volatile ingredients in a perfume.

TURNS
When a perfume turns, its color and odor changes due to oxidation as a result from exposure to air, light, and/or heat.

UNDERTONE
The subtle characteristics and nuances in a blend that present themselves in a fragrance's background. The undertone is very important to a perfume's personality.

VELVETY
A perfume that is soft and smooth, lacking harsh chemical notes.

VISCOSITY
The degree to which a fluid moves and flows under an applied force. With carrier oils, it may be noted as "thin" or "thick," etc.

VOLATILE
A substance that is unstable and evaporates easily, such an essential oil.

VOLUME
A perfume that spreads widely in the atmosphere.

WARMING
A substance that raises the temperature slightly.

WHIFF
An scent naturally given off by a composition.

WOODY
A scent that evokes freshly cut, dry wood.

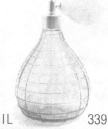

OTHER BOOKS

BY

REBECCA PARK TOTILO

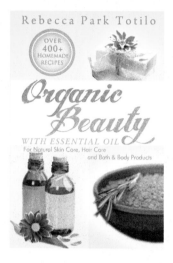

Organic Beauty With Essential Oil: Over 400+ Homemade Recipes for Natural Skin Care, Hair Care and Bath & Body Products

Sweep aside all those harmful chemically-based cosmetics and make your own organic bath and body products at home with the magic of potent essential oils! In this book, you'll find a luxurious array of over 400 Eco-friendly recipes that call for breathtaking fragrances and soothing, rich organic ingredients satisfying you head to toe. Included you'll find helpful can have the confidence knowing which essential oil to use and how much when creating your own body scrub, lip butter, or lotion bar! Discover how easy it is to make bath treats like fragrant shower gels, dreamy bubble baths, luscious creams and lotions, deep cleansing masks and facials for literally pennies using only a few essential oils and ingredients from your own kitchen with Organic Beauty with Essential Oil.

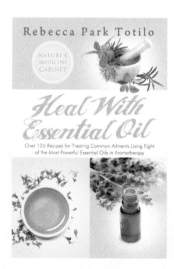

Heal With Essential Oil: Nature's Medicine Cabinet

Using essential oils drawn from nature's own medicine cabinet of flowers, trees, seeds and roots, man can tap into God's healing power to heal oneself from almost any pain. Find relief from many conditions and rejuvenate the body. With over 125 recipes, this practical guide will walk you through in the most easy-to-understand form how to treat common ailments with your essential oils for everyday living. Filled with practical advice on therapeutic blending of oils and safety, a directory of the most effective oils for common ailments and easy to follow remedies chart, and prescriptive blends for aches, pains and sicknesses.

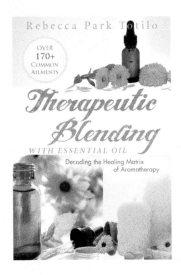

Therapeutic Blending With Essential Oil: Decoding the Healing Matrix of Aromatherapy

Therapeutic Blending With Essential Oil unlocks the healing power of essential oils and guides you through the intricate matrix of aromatherapy, with a compilation of over 170 common ailments. Discover how to properly formulate a blend for any physical or emotional symptom with easy to follow customizable recipes. Now, you can make your own personalized massage oils, hand and body lotions, bath gels, compresses, salve ointments, smelling salts, nasal inhalers and more. This exhaustive guide takes all the guesswork out of blending essential oils from how many drops to include in a blend, to working with and measuring thick oils, to how often to apply it for acute or chronic conditions. It also shows you how to create a single blend for multiple conditions. Even if you run out of oil for a favorite recipe, this book shows you how to substitute it with another oil.

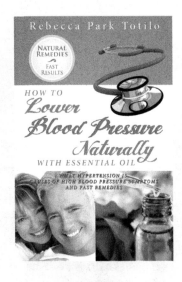

How To Lower Blood Pressure Naturally With Essential Oil: What Hypertension Is, Causes of High Pressure Symptoms and Fast Remedies

One out of three adults have it, and another one-third don't realize it. Oftentimes, it goes undetected for years. Even those who take multiple medications for it still don't have it under control. It's no secret -- high blood pressure is rampant in America. High blood pressure, or hypertension, has become a household term. Between balancing meds and monitoring diets though, are the true causes -- and best treatments -- hidden in the shadows? In How to Lower Blood Pressure Naturally With Essential Oil, Rebecca Park Totilo sheds light on what high blood pressure is, the causes and symptoms of high blood pressure, and which essential oils regulate blood pressure and how to use essential oils as a natural, alternative method.

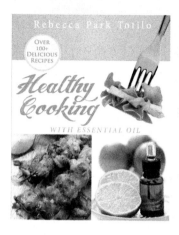

Healthy Cooking with Essential Oil

Imagine transforming an everyday dish into something extraordinary using only a drop or two of essential oil can enliven everything from soups, salads, to main dishes and desserts. Boasting flavor and fragrance, these intense essences can turn a dull, boring meal into something appetizing and delicious. Essential oils are fun, easy-to-use and beneficial, compared to the traditional stale, dried herbs and spices found in most pantries today. Healthy food should never be thought of as mere fuel for the body, it should be enjoyed as a multi-sensory experience that brings therapeutic value as well as nourishment. For years we have limited the use of essential oils to scented candles and soaps, in the belief that they were unsafe to consume (and some are!). However, more people are realizing the value of using pure essential oils to enhance their diet. In Healthy Cooking With Essential Oil, you will learn how cooking with essential oils can open up a wealth of creative opportunities in the kitchen.

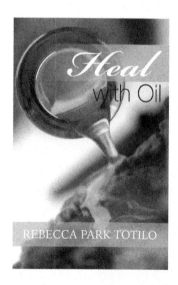

Heal With Oil: How to Use the Essential Oils of Ancient Scripture

During ancient times, spices, resins and other aromatics were an integral part of the Hebraic culture. People of the Holy Land understood the use of fragrant plants in maintaining wellness and physical healing, as well as the plant's oil to enhance their spiritual state in worship, prayer and confession, and for cleansing and purification from sin. Since the creation, fragrant oils have been inhaled, applied to the body, and taken internally in which the benefits extended to every aspect of their being. Buried within the passages of scriptures lies a hidden treasure - possibly every man's answer to illness and disease. Now you can learn their secret and discover how to transform your life and walk in divine health.

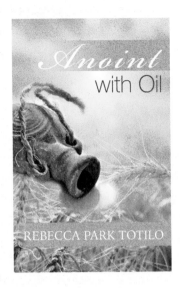

Anoint with Oil

If you were taught by church leaders that anointing with oil ceased during Old Testament times, or that it is simply "symbolic" and has no power or significance today, you may be missing beauty and depth in your spiritual journey. Anointing with oil brings real benefits into your life, such as promotion, discernment, sensitivity, fruitfulness, and declaration. In Anoint With Oil, Rebecca Park Totilo shares an aromatic and sacred expedition through the scriptures, showing the purpose of anointing with oil, the methods used in the Bible and their symbolism, the ingredients of the holy anointing oil, and the uses of essential oils mentioned in the Old and New Testaments. Discover new scents within these pages and find out: - Why the right ear, right thumb, and right big toe? - What is the mysterious fifth ingredient of the holy anointing oil? - Which oils did Jesus anoint with? - Who performs the anointing ritual? - How can I benefit from anointing with oil?

CPSIA information can be obtained
at www.ICGtesting.com
Printed in the USA
LVOW06s2316291217
561303LV00006B/6/P